This book has been sponsored by Ethicon Endo-Surgery (Europe) GmbH and Johnson & Johnson MEDICAL GmbH, Norderstedt, Germany. The authors are responsible for the content of the publication. Information provided in this book is offered in good faith as an educational tool for health care professionals. The information has been thoroughly reviewed and is believed to be useful and accurate at the time of its publication, but is offered without warranty of any kind. The authors and the sponsors shall not be responsible for any loss or damage arising from its use. Always refer to the instructions for use that comes with each device for the most current and complete instructions.

OPERATION PRIMER volume 9

Laparoscopic Gastric Bypass

Editors

Marc Immenroth
Jürgen Brenner

Authors

Hans Lönroth
Karl Miller

assisted by

Indre Offermann

Maike Aukstinnis
Ann-Katrin Güler
Astrid Künemund
Annegret Röhling
Detlev Ruge

Springer

Authors

Hans Lönroth, M.D., PhD
Associate Professor of Surgery, Head of the Surgical Department, Sahlgrenska University Hospital,
413 45 Göteborg, Sweden

Karl Miller, M.D., FACS
Associate Professor of Surgery, Head of the Surgical Department, Krankenhaus Hallein,
Bürgermeisterstr. 34,
5400 Hallein, Austria

Editors

Marc Immenroth, PhD
Senior Marketing Manager EP Germany & Plus Platform & Synthetic Absorbables D-A-CH,
Johnson & Johnson MEDICAL GmbH,
Robert-Koch-Straße 1,
22851 Norderstedt, Germany

Jürgen Brenner, MD
Managing Director
Eric Krauthammer & Dr. Jürgen Brenner
Creative Team-Leadership

ISBN 978-3-642-23001-1 Laparoscopic Gastric Bypass

Bibliografische Information der Deutschen Bibliothek
The Deutsche Bibliothek lists this publication in Deutsche Nationalbibliographie;
detailed bibliographic data are available in the internet at http://dnb.ddb.de.

First published in Germany in 2012 by Springer Medizin Verlag
springer.com

SPIN 80083501
Layout and typesetting: Dr. Carl GmbH, Stuttgart, Germany
Printing: Stürtz GmbH, Würzburg, Germany

18/5135/DK – 5 4 3 2 1 0

EDITORS' PREFACE

What drives us to further pursue the Operation Primer series?

It is the grateful patients to which our efforts are dedicated. We have proven that when correctly applied, the nodal point method increases the confidence of the surgeon and with this; patient operation results are significantly improved.

This is the motivation of us and the authors!

With the current Operation Primer, we are adding another important component to the individual therapy of morbidly obese patients. We consider ourselves lucky to have had *Hans Lönroth* of Sweden and *Karl Miller* of Austria join us; two surgeons who engaged themselves with fervor and professional ability.

The Operation Primer should help to prepare oneself, especially for that which can unexpectedly occur. They should assist in learning and the safe implementation of the skills learned.

We can not say what influence future technical developments will have, but adequate preparation for what may come, including systematic learning with the help of mental training, is an excellent method. Studying and mental training determine the performance results in the practical implementation on the patient, leading to more successful operations.

Experts in the field of bariatrics, *Hans Lönroth* and *Karl Miller,* have worked to develop this Operation Primer in accordance with the mental training methods which are a staple of previous editions. Each nodal point has been carefully and collaboratively defined and is aligned with the most sensible course of action; these points should be consecutively observed.

We have also received excellent support from *Dr. Carl GmbH,* which has accompanied us at each stage of the working process and has contributed greatly to making these innovative surgical textbooks what they are. The diagrams, line drawings, etc. were produced mainly by *Thomas Heller.* The existing concept of practical surgical primers has become reality through the publishing company *Springer Medizin Verlag Heidelberg.* Sincere thanks to all of them.

Above all else, patient safety is our main aim, and we hope that our books will assist the reader in achieving this goal.

Wladimir Horowitz once said: „If I don't practice for a day, I know it. If I don't practice for two days, the critics know it. If I don't practice for three days, the audience knows it."

The Editors January 2012

AUTHORS' PREFACE

The problems related to obesity are today well known and the co-morbidities well documented. Still, the incidence and prevalence of obesity is increasing all over the world. Surgery as a solution is widely debated, but we are still waiting for non-surgical solutions that can compete with the outcome of surgery. Obesity surgery has been practiced for more than 50 years and already in the 1960's Mason and Griffen presented gastric bypass as a well functioning operation for weight reduction. The gastric bypass performed today is, for the most part, the same operation, but with modifications and new technical solutions aimed to optimize the outcome and reduce adverse effects of surgery. This book aims to describe two techniques of gastric bypass. The design is based on evidence from literature and the authors' personal preference related to instruments and tools to simplify the operation. Without a doubt, the laparoscopic technique in performing obesity surgery has increased the popularity of this treatment solution. Laparoscopic surgery may be technically demanding at some points, but it also enables us to document the operations through video and share our knowledge with others. Hopefully this presentation will help you as a surgeon to avoid mistakes already made by others.

Hans Lönroth
Karl Miller

January 2012

The beneficial effects of modest weight loss have been widely accepted since the Goldstein review was published in 1992.

In the World Health Organization (WHO) report on obesity, published in the year 2000, it was estimated that a 10 kg weight loss was associated with 10 and 20 mmHg reductions in systolic and diastolic blood pressure, respectively, 10–15 % reductions in total and low-density lipoprotein cholesterol, 30 % reduction in triglycerides and an 8 % increase in high-density lipoprotein (HDL) cholesterol. However, the incidence of obesity is growing dramatically in the world and therefore the number of surgical interventions in the field of obesity surgery is increasing.

The Roux-en-Y gastric bypass has become the gold standard in different regions of the world and is more frequently classified as a metabolic surgery, as several studies could show enormous benefits regarding not only weight loss, but additional side-effects like type 2 diabetes, hypertension, hyperlipidemia among others. The recently published IDF Statement (IDF-International Diabetes Federation) stated that metabolic surgery is currently the only effective treatment for type 2 diabetes and its co-morbidities. Moreover, the Roux-en-Y gastric bypass is a sufficient therapeutical option in the treatment of acid reflux (GERD) and the prevention and treatment of Barrets esophagitis.

Multiple long-term studies have shown that the positive effects on weight and diabetes are persistent and the side-effects regarding the malabsorption of fat-soluble vitamins and vitamin B_{12} are small in the case of sufficient postoperative vitamin substitution. In experienced hands, Roux-en-Y gastric bypass has shown to be safe in comparison to other bariatric procedures and to create less post-operative complications than other procedures like sleeve gastrectomy and biliopancreatic diversion.

Long-term weight loss with more than 60 % of excess body weight after gastric bypass has shown the efficiency of the procedure in the treatment of the potentially life-threatening metabolic syndrome in the long and short term.

Regarding the increasing incidence of obesity worldwide the estimated number of surgical interventions is dramatically growing. Procedures with positive long-term effects such as the gastric bypass can be expected to keep their primary position within the numbers of surgical procedures.

Moreover, the Roux-en-Y gastric bypass is one of the most widely used secondary/revisional procedures. It is a standard in the laparoscopic approach and is currently also being developed for less invasive methods like single port or incisionless procedures.

Rudolf A. Weiner

President EU-Chapter of IFSO
President XVI World Congress IFSO 2011

January 2012

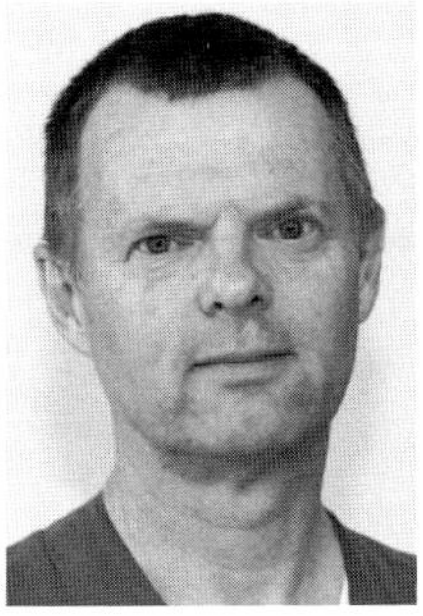

Hans H. Lönroth, M.D., PhD

- Studied medicine at Karolinska Institute, Stockholm, Sweden
- 1977 MD Karolinska Institute, Stockholm, Sweden
- 1985 Qualified as a General Surgeon Sahlgrenska University Hospital, Gothenburg, Sweden
- 1990 PhD Medical Sience Sahlgrenska Academy, Gothenburg, Sweden
- 1995 Associate Professor of Surgery at Sahlgrenska Academy, University of Gothenburg, Sweden
- Since 2005 Head of Department of Surgery at Sahlgrenska University Hospital Gothenburg, Sweden

Focus of Research and Work

- Upper gastrointestinal surgery
- Reflux esophagitis
- Bariatric surgery
- Achalasia
- Gastric pacing in gastrointestinal motor function disorders

Experience

- Laparoscopic surgery
- Development of surgical technique of vertical gastric banding, gastric bypass and gastric pacing of motor function disorders
- Since 1996 organized international workshops in bariatric surgery with main focus on gastric bypass
- Faculty in several international workshops and meetings since 1995

Memberships

- Swedish Surgical Society
- Swedish Society of Laparoscopic Surgery
- Nordic Surgical Society
- EAES (European Association of Endoscopic Surgeons)
- IFSO (International Federation for the Surgery of Obesity and related diseases)
- Editorial board member of the scientific journal *Obesity Surgery*
- Referee of the *British Journal of Surgery*

Author of many scientific articles and peer-reviewed publications in surgical journals

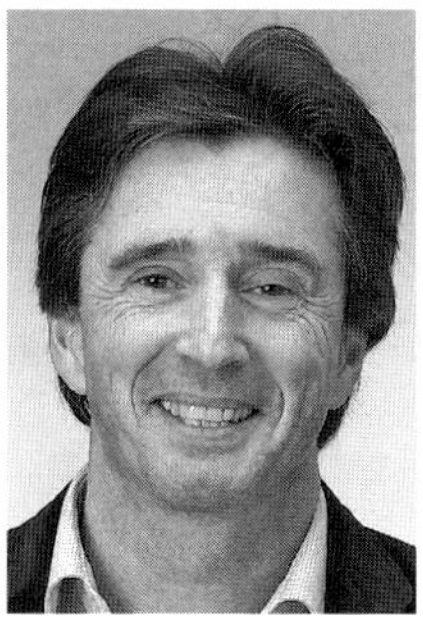

Karl Miller, M.D., FACS

- Studied medicine in Innsbruck, Austria
- 1983 Doctorate in Medicine at the University of Innsbruck, Austria
- 1991 Qualified as General Surgeon
- 1995–2000 Vice Chief at the 2nd Surgical Department of the General Hospital Salzburg, Austria
- 1996 Associate Professor of Surgery at the University of Innsbruck, Austria
- Since 1996 Faculty of the European Surgical Institute in Norderstedt, Germany
- Since 2001 Head of the Surgical Department of the Hospital Hallein, Austria
- Since 2003 Associate Editor of the Journal *Obesity Surgery*
- Since 2008 Associate Editor of the *European Journal of Obesity*
- 2010–2011 President of the International Federation for the Surgery of Obesity and Metabolic Disorders (IFSO)
- Since 2011 Editorial Board Member of Bariatric Times
- Since 2012 Editorial Board Member of the Journal Surgery of Obesity and Metabolic Disorders (SOARD)

Focus of Research and Work
- Bariatric surgery
- Surgical education

Experience
- Developed and standardized the surgical technique for laparoscopic gastric banding (Pars flaccida technique)
- Experienced in laparoscopic gastric surgery and laparoscopic functional surgery of the stomach (Nissen and Toupet fundoplicatio)
- Since 2003 organized 20 international workshops per year where more than 650 surgeons worldwide were given „hands-on" training in laparoscopic gastric banding and gastric bypass
- 1999 Organized the World Congress on Obesity Surgery in Salzburg, Austria

Author of many scientific articles published in surgical journals

Contents

Appendices

Introduction

From an educational point of view, the Operation Primer is somewhat plagiaristic. The layout – and this can be admitted freely – is taken over largely from commonly available cook books. In such books, the ingredients and cooking utensils required to prepare the recipe in question are normally listed first. The most important cooking procedures are then described briefly in the text. Photographs support the written explanations and show what the dish should look like when prepared. Sometimes diagrams and illustrations make individual cooking steps clearer.

Despite these obvious parallels, there is a crucial difference between cook books and the Operation Primer: in the Operation Primer, complicated and complex surgical techniques are described that are intended to help the surgeon and his team perform an operation safely and economically. Ultimately, it always comes down to the patient's welfare. The following must therefore be said early in this introduction:

- The use of the Operation Primer as an aid to operating requires that surgical techniques have first been completely mastered.
- Being alert to possible mistakes is categorically the most important principle when operating; avoiding mistakes is crucial.

The concept of the Operation Primer originated in a scientific study with the title "Mental Training in Surgical Education" that formed part of a collaborative project between the surgical department of the University of Cologne (under Prof. Hans Troidl), the Institute of Sports and Sports Science of the University of Heidelberg, and the European Surgical Institute (ESI) in Norderstedt. Laparoscopic cholecystectomy was the initial focus.

Mental training is derived from top-class sports. This is understood as methodically repeating and consciously imagining actions and movements without actually carrying them out at the same time (cf. Driskell, Copper & Moran, 1994; Feltz & Landers, 1983; Immenroth, 2003; Immenroth, Eberspächer & Hermann, 2008). Scientific involvement with imagining movement has a long tradition in medical and psychological research. As early as 1852, Lotze described how imagining and perceiving movements can lead to a concurrent performance "with quiet movements …" (Lotze, 1852). This phenomenon later became known by the names "Ideomotion" and "Carpenter effect" (Carpenter, 1874).

In the collaborative project, mental training was modified in such a way that it could be employed in the training and further education of young surgeons. In mental training in surgery, surgeons visualize the operation from the inner perspective without performing any actual movements, i.e., they go through the operation step by step in their mind's eye. In the study that was conducted at the ESI, the first Operation Primer was used as the basis for this visualization. In this primer, laparoscopic cholecystectomy was subdivided into individual, clearly depicted steps, the so-called nodal points.

The study evaluated the effect of the mental training on learning laparoscopic cholecystectomy compared with practical training and with a control group. The planning, conduct, and evaluation of the study took 7 years (2000–2007), with over 100 surgeons participating.

The results corresponded exactly with the expectations: the mentally trained surgeons improved in a similar degree to those surgeons who received additional practical training on a pelvi trainer simulator (in some subscales even more). Moreover, there was greater improvement in these two groups compared with the control group, which did not receive any additional mental or practical training (cf. in detail, Immenroth, Bürger, Brenner, Nagelschmidt, Eberspächer & Troidl, 2007; Immenroth, Bürger, Brenner, Kemmler, Nagelschmidt, Eberspächer & Troidl, 2005; Immenroth, Eberspächer, Nagelschmidt, Troidl, Bürger, Brenner, Berg, Müller & Kemmler, 2005).

Recently, a significant improvement in surgical knowledge and confidence was shown by both experienced and novice surgeons in another study about mental training in laparoscopic surgery (Arora et al., 2010). Therefore, mental training can be seen as a cost- and time-effective training tool that should be integrated into surgical training.

Furthermore, the study by Immenroth et al. (2007) included a questionnaire to determine the extent to which the mentally trained surgeons accepted mental training as a teaching method in surgery. Mental training was assessed as very positive by all 34 mentally trained surgeons. The Operation Primer received particular acclaim in the evaluation:

- 82 % of the surgeons wished to use similar self-made Operation Primers in their daily work.
- 85 % of the surgeons attributed the success of the mental training at least in part to the Operation Primer.
- 88 % of the surgeons wanted to have these Operation Primers as a fixed component of the course at the ESI.

This positive response to the study was the starting point for the production of the present series of Operation Primers.

Prior to publication, the Operation Primer was developed by methodical and didactical means and then adapted to the readers' needs and wishes. This was carried out following a survey of 93 surgeons (interns, resident doctors, assistant medical directors and medical directors) who participated in surgical courses at the ESI. They evaluated in detail the structure and components by means of a questionnaire.

The results of this survey gave important findings on how to optimize the Operation Primer. The sense and representation of the nodal points, the comprehensibility and detail of the text, and the photographs of the operation were highly valued especially by young surgeons (Güler, Immenroth, Berg, Bürger & Gawad, 2006). The comprehensive research undertaken with this Operation Primer series will ensure its overall value to the reader.

Structure and handling of the Operation Primer

In the present series of Operation Primers, an attempt has been made to standardize the described laparoscopic operations as much as possible. This is achieved first by applying the same format to all operating techniques described. Second, operative sequences that are performed identically in all operations are always explained using the same blocks of text. By following a general structure for the description of all operations and by using identical text blocks, it was intended to aid recognition of recurring patterns and their translation into action even for different operations.

I Preparations for the operation
II Creating the pneumoperitoneum – placing the trocar for the scope
III Placing the working trocars
IV Nodal points
V Management of difficult situations and complications
Appendices

The Operation Primer is divided into five chapters, each identified by Roman numerals and different register colors in the margin. The contents of the individual chapters will now be explained.

In **Preparations for the operation**, the basic instruments for all laparoscopic operations and then the additional instruments for the specific operation are listed. This is followed by a detailed description of the positioning and shaving of the patient, attaching the dispersive electrode, setting up the equipment, skin disinfection and sterile draping of the patient. The operative preparation is concluded with a detailed description and an illustration of how the operating team is to be positioned for the operation in question.

3 possibilities for creating the pneumoperitoneum: the choice is up to the surgeon

Veress needle = greatest danger!

In the chapter **Creating the pneumoperitoneum – placing the trocar for the scope**, three alternatives are shown in detail: the Hasson method, trocar with optical obturator, and Veress needle. The choice of method is up to the individual surgeon. All three alternatives are employed in surgical practice. However, it should be pointed out that the greatest danger in minimally invasive surgery is the insertion of the Veress needle, as it is done "blind".

Continuous illustration of the trocar positions

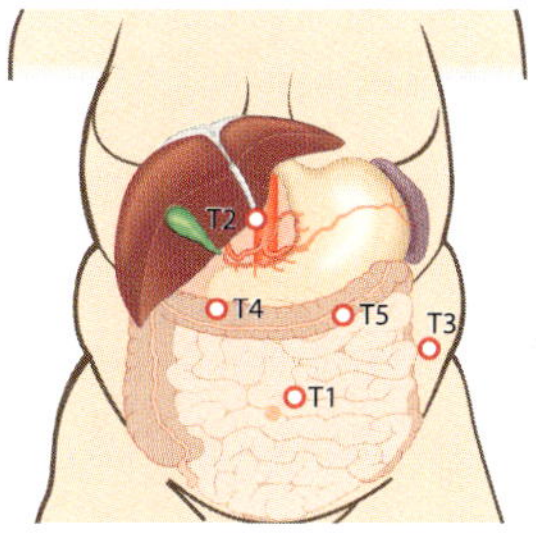

Placing the working trocars is explained in detail in the next chapter. The written explanations are supplemented by a diagram. In order to keep a constant overview of the placement of the trocars, even during the following description of the operation sequence, this illustration is shown in diminished size in every single operative step.

Nodal point = term from top-class sports

Nodal points:
1) absolutely essential
2) successive order
3) no degrees of freedom

The core of the Operation Primer is the chapter **Nodal points**. This is where the actual sequence of the operation is described in detail. However, prior to this detailed explanation, the term nodal point will be explained briefly. In the Editors' preface and introduction, mental training was mentioned as a form of training used successfully in top-class sports for decades, and this is where the term originates. In sports as in surgery, a nodal point is understood as one of those structural components of movement that are absolutely essential for performing the movement optimally. Nodal points have to be passed through in succession and are characterized by a reduction in the degrees of freedom of action. In mental training they act as orientation points for methodical repetition and conscious imagining of the athletic or operative movement (cf. in detail Immenroth et al., 2008).

Flow chart of the sequence of nodal points on each double page

For every operation in the Operation Primer series, these nodal points were extracted in a prolonged process by the authors in collaboration with the editors. The nodal points represent the basic structural framework of an operation. Because of their particular relevance and for better orientation, all of the nodal points in the Operation Primer are shown on the left on each double page as a flow chart. The current nodal point is highlighted graphically. The instruments required for this nodal point and the specific trocars for it are listed in a box on the right, beside the flow chart.

Maximum of 7±2 instructions per nodal point

Below the instrument box, instructions regarding the nodal point are given as briefly as possible. According to Miller (1956), people can best store 7±2 units of information ("Magical number 7"). Therefore, no more than seven single instructions are listed per nodal point, if possible. With regard to the instructions, it should be noted that the change of instruments between the individual nodal points is not described explicitly as a rule; rather, this is apparent through different instruments in the instrument box.

Watch-outs are pointed out in red!

Where necessary, particular moments where special attention is needed are pointed out in red.

Alternatives: In small blue print at the end of the nodal point.

The described operation sequence is only one way of performing the operation safely and economically, namely the way preferred by the authors. Undoubtedly, a number of other equally valid operation sequences exist. As far as possible, notes on alternative methods are given in small blue print at the end of each nodal point.

In the fifth chapter, the **Management of difficult situations and complications** is described in detail. In general, details on adhesions, bleeding, injuries to organs, etc. are given first.

Illustration of anatomical variations, an example of an operation note, details about the circular stapler technique, postoperative management, and postoperative complications in the appendices

In the **Appendices** relevant anatomical variations which can occur in the operation sequence and may require a different approach are described first. In order to give the Operation Primer even more practical relevance, an example of an operation note is then reproduced. The appendices also contain helpful hints for using a circular stapler as a variation of the gastric bypass procedure, detailed information about the postoperative management, postoperative complications and their management, as well as the bibliographical references and list of keywords.

In order to avoid repetition, reference is made throughout the text to relevant chapters of the Operation Primer, if necessary. To do this, the Roman numeral of the chapter and the number of the corresponding section are shown in parentheses. Referral is made most often to the fifth chapter, where the management of difficult situations and complications is described. These references are set off in red letters.

(→ p. 64, V-4) = reference to the 4th section of chapter V

All sources in the literature are listed in the bibliography

Finally, it must be pointed out that for better readability of the Operation Primer no bibliographical references at all are given in the text. However, in order to give an overview of the basic and more extensive sources, the entire literature is listed in the bibliography.

Make sure that the following preoperative requirements for laparoscopic gastric bypass have been met:

- The indication for the operation is correct.
- The patient has given detailed informed written consent.
- The bowel is prepared appropriately prior to laparoscopic gastrointestinal surgery.
- Thromboprophylaxis (low-molecular-weight heparin) has been given as per local practice.
- Single-dose perioperative antibiotic prophylaxis has been given.

Basic instruments

- Size 11 scalpel
- 10 ml syringe with 0.9 % NaCl solution
- Dissecting scissors
- 2 Langenbeck hooks
- Suction device
- Needle holder
- Suture scissors
- 2 surgical forceps
- 2 Backhaus clamps
- Compresses
- Swabs with an integral X-ray contrast strip
- Sutures:
  - Fascia: 2–0 absorbable, polyfilament
  - Subcutaneous: 3–0 absorbable, polyfilament, if necessary
  - Skin: 4–0 or 5-0 absorbable, monofilament
  - Ileum/stomach: 3–0 absorbable, mono- or polyfilament
- Trocar side closure device, if necessary
- Skin adhesive, if necessary
- Dressings

Instruments for the first access, depending on the type of access:

a) Hasson method:
- Hasson trocar (10/12 mm)
- 2 stay sutures (2–0)
- Purse-string suture (2–0)

b) Trocar with optical obturator (e.g. ENDOPATH® XCEL™ bladeless trocar, Ethicon Endo-Surgery)

c) Veress needle (e.g. ENDOPATH® Ultra Veress Insufflation Needle, Ethicon Endo-Surgery)

There should always be a basic laparotomy set in the operating room so that in an emergency a laparotomy can be performed without delay!

Alternative: The usage of antibacterial suture material coated with Triclosan, the Plus Suture generation from Ethicon, is also recommended.

Additional instruments for laparoscopic gastric bypass

Trocars:	(e.g. ENDOPATH® XCEL™ trocar, Ethicon Endo-Surgery)
T1: Trocar for the scope	(10/12 mm)
T2: Working trocar	(5 mm or 10/12 mm; depending on the liver retracting device)
T3: Working trocar	(5 mm or 10/12 mm)
T4: Working trocar	(10/12 mm)
T5: Working trocar	(10/12 mm)

- Additional trocars, if necessary
- Reducer caps, if necessary
- Angled scope (0° scope, if necessary, for trocar with optical obturator)

Extra-long trocars are usually not required. The only instrument that should always be extra-long is the HF (high frequency) hook!

- Liver retracting device with fixation arm
- Additional liver retracting device with fixation arm, if necessary
- Extra-long HF (high-frequency) electrode handle and hook
- Ultrasonic device (e.g. Harmonic® shears, Ethicon Endo-Surgery)

Before using Harmonic® instruments read the instructions for use and become familiar with the instrument!

- Endoscopic linear cutter (e.g. Echelon Flex™ ENDOPATH® Stapler, articulating endoscopic linear cutter 45 mm, Ethicon Endo-Surgery)
- Different cartridges (depending on tissue thickness)
- Curved dissector
- 2 atraumatic grasping forceps (5 mm and/or 10 mm)
- Atraumatic grasping forceps with landmark, e.g. Babcock clamp with landmark (5 mm and/or 10 mm)
- Dissecting swab
- Curved scissors
- Needle holder
- Sutures
- Clip applier (e.g. LAPRA-TY® clip applier, Ethicon Products)
- Suture clips (e.g. LAPRA-TY® suture clips, Ethicon Products)
- Suction-irrigation instrument

For the anesthetist:

- 5 ml methylene blue 1 %
- 10 ml syringe with cannula
- Small bowl

Always refer to the instructions for use that comes with each device for the most current and complete instructions.

Basic instruments

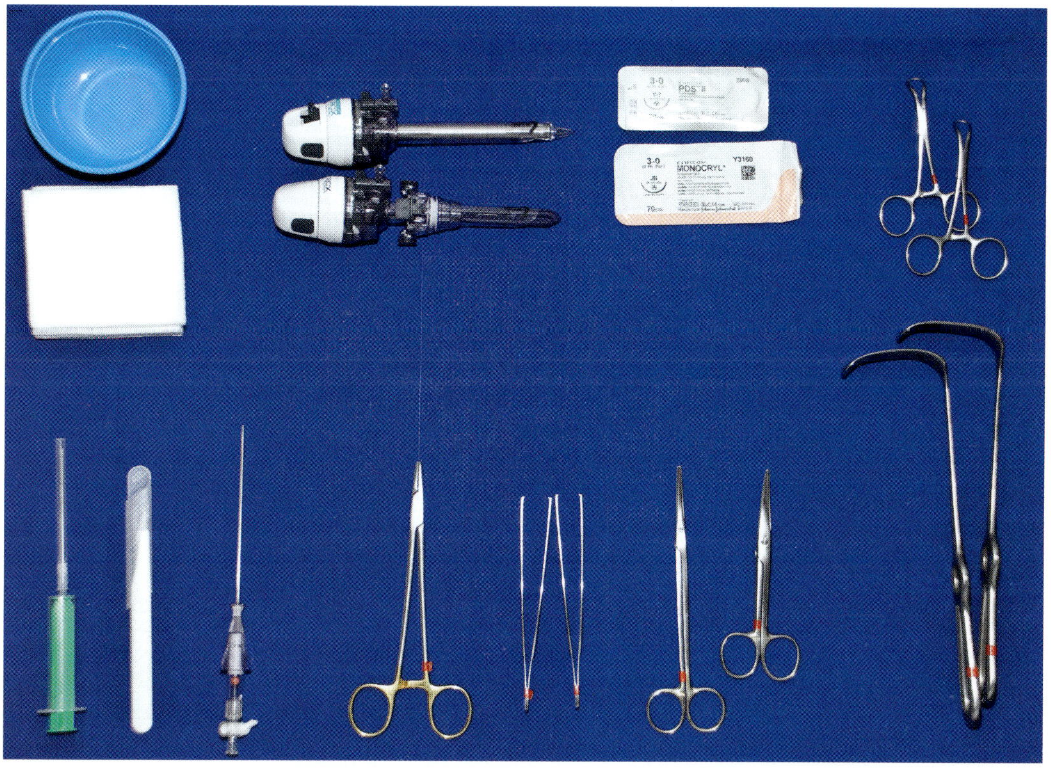

Additional instruments for laparoscopic gastric bypass

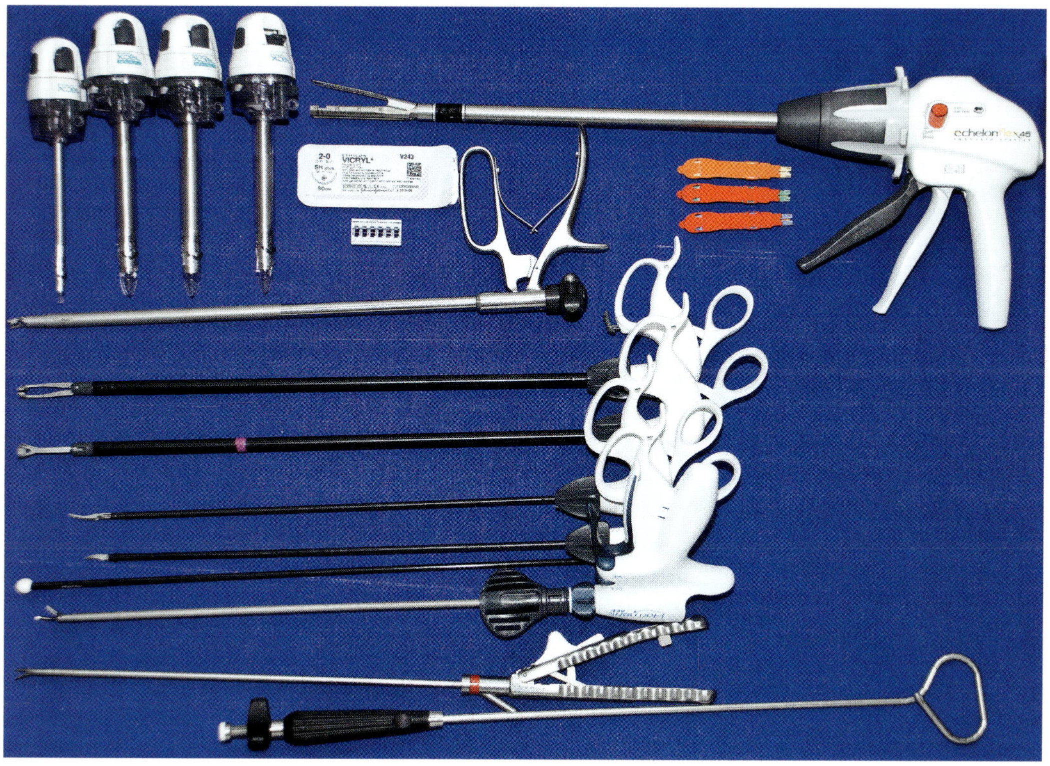

Emptying the urinary bladder

- In order to achieve an excellent exposure into the small pelvis and to avoid injuries to the urinary bladder, make sure that the patient's bladder is emptied preoperatively by placing a temporary transurethral catheter.

Positioning of the patient

The technical fittings, especially the operating table, must be approved and functional for the patient's weight!

- Position the patient in lithotomy position.
- Stretch thighs and legs apart with a slight flexure.
- Place both arms at an angle not greater than 70° to the long axis of the body in order to avoid injuries to the axillary nerve.
- Pad the shoulder, elbow and knee joints in order to avoid pressure injuries, particularly of the nerves.
- For better positioning of the patient, hyperextend the back in the lumbar region by means of a pad or by appropriate adjustment of the operating table.
- Use a padded board as a surface to lie on to prevent the patient from sliding when put in extreme positions.
- After creating the pneumoperitoneum and inserting the trocar for the scope (→ p. 25, II) and the scope (→ p. 30, III), put the patient in a reverse Trendelenburg position (30°).

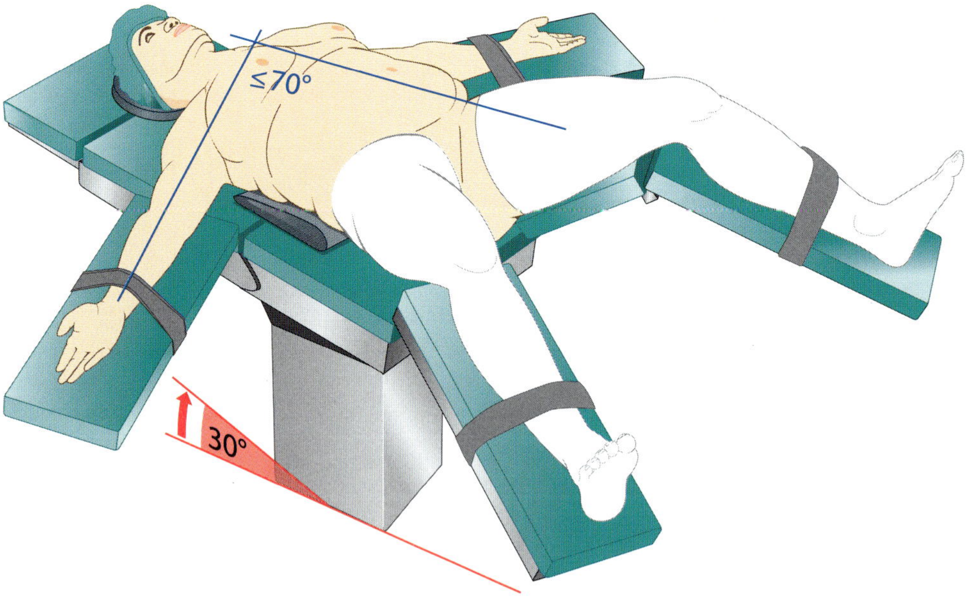

Shaving

- Shave the patient from the mamillae to above the pubic symphysis and from the left to the right anterior superior iliac spine in order to be able to convert to a conventional operation if complications occur.
- If monopolar current is used, shave the application site of the dispersive electrode (as close as possible to the operating field, e.g. on the upper thigh).

Alternative: Instead of shaving, the hair can be removed by cutting off with scissors or with depilatory cream.

Dispersive electrode

- Before placing the dispersive electrode, ensure that the skin at this site and all skin areas in contact with the table are absolutely dry.
- Then stick the entire surface of the electrode carefully above the greatest possible muscle mass (e.g. on the upper thigh). The conducting cable must be at the greatest possible distance from the operating field.

When using monopolar current, always guard against burns on moist areas of the skin due to current!

Skin disinfection

- Disinfect the skin from the mamillae to the pubic symphysis. Pay particular attention to careful disinfection of all skin folds.

Sterile draping

- Drape the operating field with sterile drapes so that it is limited cranially at the level of the xiphoid, just above the umbilicus caudally, and by the midaxillary lines laterally.
- During sterile draping of the operating field, position the fixation arm of the liver retracting device at the right side of the table at the level of the liver.

Setting up the equipment

- Set the generators of the Harmonic® shears and of the HF electrode to an appropriate power level for the intended use.
- Position the foot pedals, if used.
- Attach the suction-irrigation instrument.
- Select a maximum pressure of 12 mmHg on the CO_2 insufflator (with a flow of 6–8 l/min).

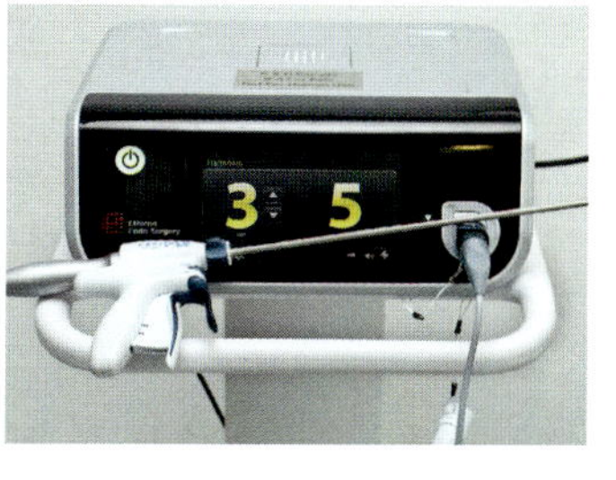

Generator GEN11 for Harmonic® shears (Ethicon Endo-Surgery)

Positioning of the operating team

- The surgeon stands between the patient's spread legs.
- The camera assistant stands to the left at the level of the patient's pelvis.
- The scrub nurse stands to the right, at the level of the patient's knee.
- The monitor is located in the line of vision of the surgeon and the camera assistant, hanging behind the patient's head.

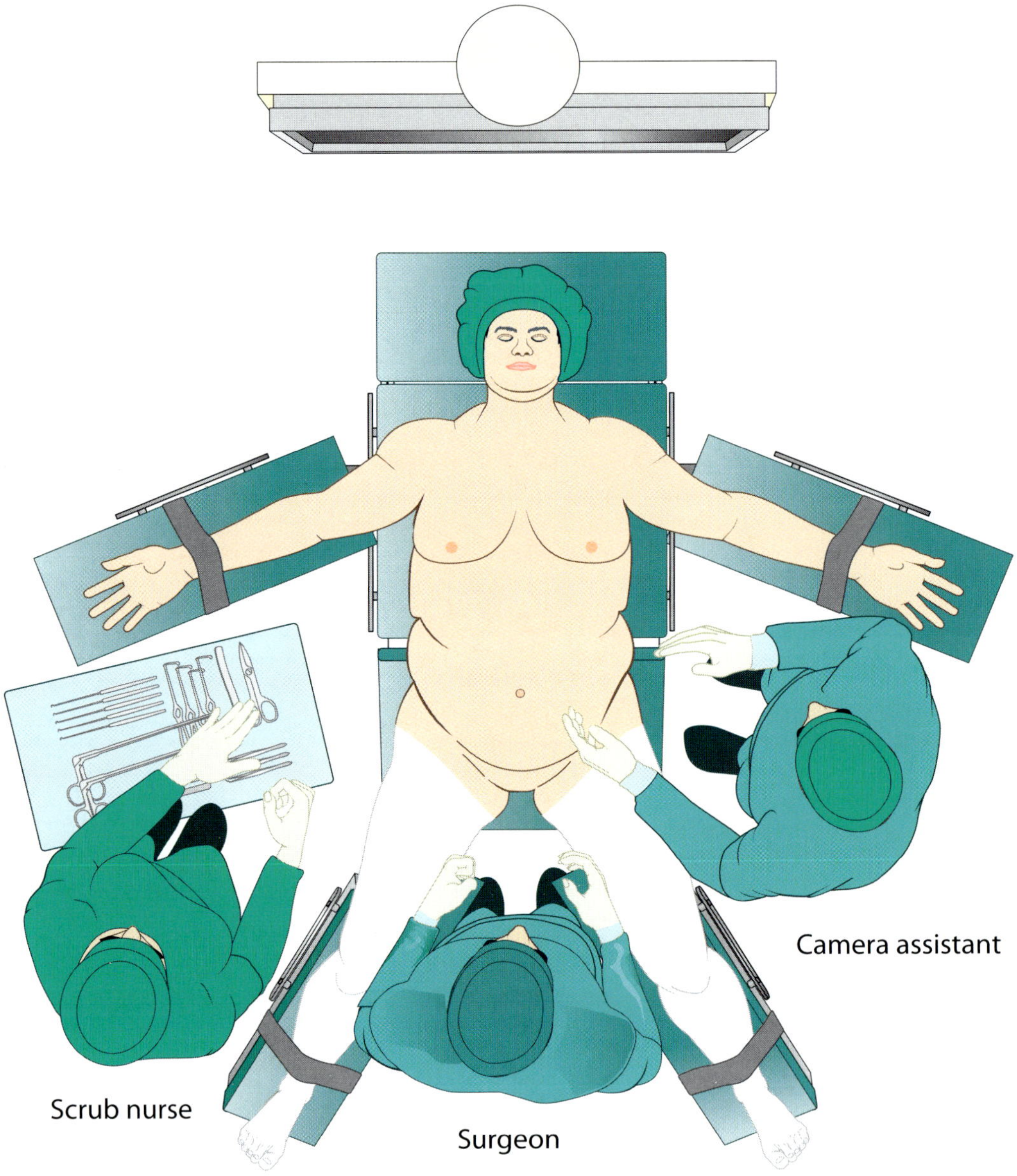

Alternative: If a ceiling monitor is not available, position the monitor in the line of vision of the surgeon and the camera assistant on the right at the level of the patient's head.

Alternative: The surgeon stands on the patient´s right side with the patient´s legs together. The camera assistant stands to the left.

Creating the pneumoperitoneum – placing the trocar for the scope

There are three ways of creating a pneumoperitoneum, which will be described in detail below:

a) Hasson method (open technique)

b) Trocar with optical obturator

c) Veress needle (closed technique)

Because of the large variety of trocars available and the resulting variety of methods of introducing the trocars, follow their individual instruction manuals!

Note the following special features when creating the pneumoperitoneum in laparoscopic obesity surgery:

- **The thickness of the abdominal wall may require a larger incision, which may make gas-proof placement of the Hasson trocar difficult (→ p. 26, IIa)!**
- **Use of an optical obturator in the trocar has proven to be helpful in obesity surgery (→ p. 27, IIb)!**
- **Select the access for the Veress needle in the left upper abdomen in order to minimize the injury risk of patients with hepatomegaly (→ p. 28, IIc)!**
- **The resting intra-abdominal pressure is often increased up to 8–9 mmHg in obese patients!**

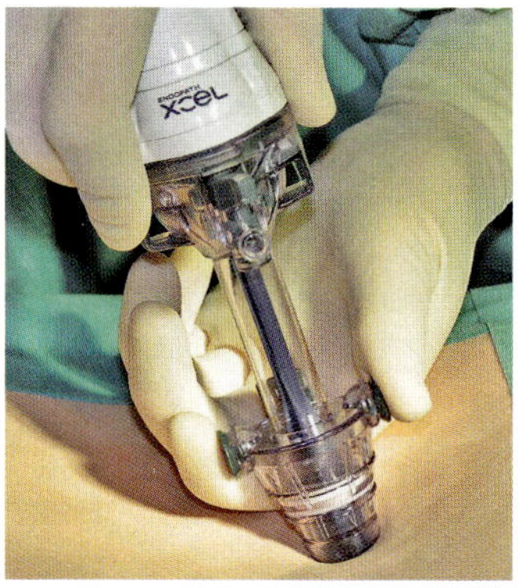

a) Hasson method (open technique)

Size 11 scalpel
Scissors
2 surgical forceps
2 Langenbeck hooks
2 stay sutures (2–0)
Purse-string suture (2–0)
Hasson trocar (10/12 mm)

In obese patients, the use of the Hasson technique can be very difficult or even impossible!

Incise the skin about 15 cm below the xiphoid and 1–2 fingers paramedian on the left, making a 1.5–2 cm skin incision.

Ensure that the skin incision is the correct length:

- **An incision that is too small can make the insertion of the trocars much more difficult. If the skin around the trocar then suffers increased tension, this may lead to skin necrosis!**
- **An incision that is too large can result in gas loss and trocar dislocation (→ p. 64, V-4b)!**

Spread the subcutaneous fat with the scissors as far as the rectus abdominis muscle. Use two Langenbeck hooks to expose the fascia of the anterior rectus sheath.

Then insert two 2–0 stay sutures on the fascia of the anterior rectus sheath and draw the fascia upwards by pulling the sutures.

Use a scalpel to open the fascia between the two stay sutures over a distance of 1.5 cm. Then spread the rectus abdominis muscle as far as the posterior rectus sheath.

To expose the fascia of the posterior rectus sheath, retract the rectus abdominis muscle with its anterior sheath by repositioning the Langenbeck hooks.

Now lift the fascia of the posterior rectus sheath and the peritoneum with the surgical forceps and incise them with the scissors over a length of about 1–1.5 cm. Check for the presence of close adhesions by inserting a finger into the incision site and palpating over the entire 360° circumference of the site.

Place a purse-string suture around the peritoneal incision and introduce the blunt Hasson trocar through the incision into the free abdominal cavity.

Secure the trocar with the two previously placed stay sutures by tying them around the wings of the trocar cone. Tighten the purse-string suture around the Hasson trocar.

Secure the CO_2 supply tube to the trocar, remove the obturator, and insufflate the gas until the preselected maximum pressure of 12 mmHg is reached.

Alternative: It is possible to perform an open technique without using a Hasson trocar. After incising the fascia of the posterior rectus sheath and the peritoneum, place a blunt probe through the incision in the free abdominal cavity, using it as a support for the placement of the trocar for the scope under visual control.

b) Trocar with optical obturator

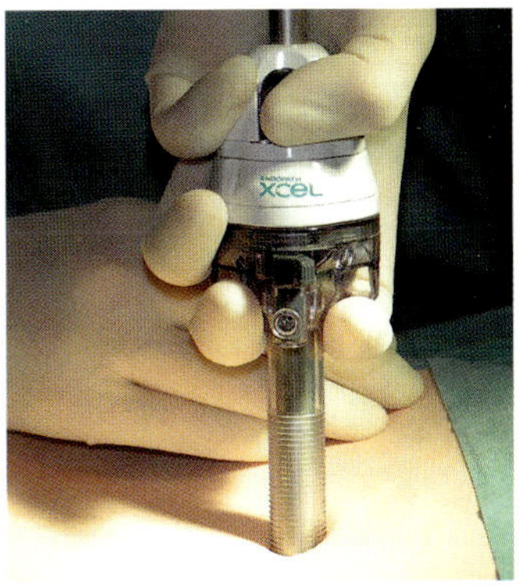

Size 11 scalpel
Trocar with optical obturator
Scope (0°)

Incise the skin about 15 cm below the xiphoid and 1–2 fingers paramedian on the left, making a 1–1.5 cm skin incision.

Ensure that the skin incision is the correct length:
- **An incision that is too small can make the insertion of the trocars much more difficult. If the skin around the trocar then suffers increased tension, this may lead to skin necrosis!**
- **An incision that is too large can result in gas loss and trocar dislocation (→ p. 64, V-4b)!**

Insert the scope into the optical obturator located in the trocar and lock the scope-locking cam.

Place the transparent conical tip into the incision. Now carefully push the different layers of the abdominal wall tangentially apart by applying light pressure and using to-and-fro rotating movements of the blunt obturator tip. The special construction of the obturator allows the layers to be identified before they are pushed apart.

Perform this tissue separation and the final perforation of the peritoneum under constant vision.

When inserting the trocar, take care
- **to go in perpendicular to the abdominal wall,**
- **to support the trocar with the hand, and**
- **not to use excessive force in order to avoid blood vessel and organ injuries in the event of loss of resistance (→ p. 63, V-2; V-3)!**

Finally, remove the scope together with the obturator from the trocar.

Secure the CO_2 supply tube to the trocar and insufflate the gas until the preselected maximum pressure of 12 mmHg is reached.

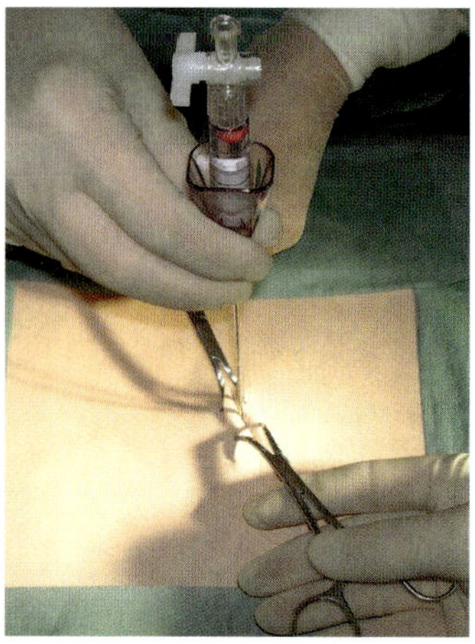

c) Veress needle (closed technique)

Insertion of the Veress needle and the first trocar are the most dangerous moments in minimally invasive surgery, as the insertion is done "blind". There are many reported cases of major injuries to the aorta and the iliac artery caused by the use of the Veress needle!

Size 11 scalpel
2 Backhaus clamps
Veress needle
10 ml syringe with NaCl solution
Trocar for the scope T1 (10/12 mm)

To minimize the risk of injury that may be caused by the Veress needle, select access in the left upper abdomen, subcostally in the midclavicular line.

In obese patients always select the access for the Veress needle in the left upper abdomen because of the usually existing hepatomegaly and the considerable amount of fatty tissue in these patients!

Patients who have undergone previous surgery carry a higher risk of having adhesions. In these patients, the Veress needle should be used with more caution!

Incise the skin about 15 cm below the xiphoid and 1–2 fingers paramedian on the left, making a 1–1.5 cm skin incision.

With the help of the assistant, elevate the abdominal wall with two Backhaus clamps, and carefully insert the Veress needle vertically, with your hand supported above the skin incision. The penetration of the abdominal wall layers by the Veress needle can be felt or even heard.

When inserting the Veress needle, take care
- **to go in perpendicular to the abdominal wall (→ p. 64, V-4a),**
- **to support the hand holding the needle, and**
- **not to use excessive force in order to avoid blood vessel and organ injuries in the event of loss of resistance (→ p. 63, V-2; V-3)!**

Check the correct position of the Veress needle by applying the following obligatory safety tests:

Aspiration test
Attach a 10 ml syringe filled with NaCl solution to the Veress needle. It should be possible to aspirate air as a sign that the intra-abdominal position is correct.

Injection test
Inject NaCl solution through the Veress needle into the abdominal cavity. This can be done easily if it is in the correct position. Increased resistance of the syringe plunger indicates a possible incorrect position of the Veress needle.

Alternative: When using the ENDOPATH® Ultra Veress Insufflation Needle (Ethicon Endo-Surgery), the valve is opened to perform the injection test, where-upon the NaCl solution is released into the abdominal cavity if the Veress needle is in the correct position. In addition, the red marker ball drops down, indicating that NaCl solution is being released into the abdominal cavity.

Rotation test

Carefully rotate the slightly tilted needle inside the abdominal cavity. If the needle can be rotated freely, adhesions in close proximity are unlikely.

Slurp test

Notice that the slurp test is hardly feasible in case of pronounced obesity!

Apply one drop of NaCl solution onto the cone of the Veress needle, placing it convex on the opening. Now pull up the abdominal wall, making sure not to fix the Veress needle with your hand. Elevating the abdominal wall will create a partial vacuum, which in turn will cause the drop of NaCl to be sucked into the abdominal cavity, provided the Veress needle is correctly placed. A substantial vacuum will cause an additional "slurping" sound to be heard at the cone of the Veress needle.

If the safety tests indicate that the Veress needle has been placed correctly, attach the gas supply tube.

Excessively high intra-abdominal resting pressure and no flow indicate that the tip of the Veress needle is obstructed, e.g. by the greater omentum (→ p. 63, V-3a). In this case, perform the following test:

Manometer test

In order to release the Veress needle, manually lift up the abdominal wall. This should result in an obvious pressure drop. If this is not the case, remove the Veress needle and then place it again.

Notice that in obese patients the resting intra-abdominal pressure is often increased up to 8–9 mmHg!

Insufflate the CO_2 until the preselected maximum pressure of 12 mmHg is reached (recommended maximum flow through the Veress needle: ~1.8 l/min). After that, remove the Veress needle from the skin incision.

To be sure that the Veress needle has been placed correctly, check for an adequate flow during the CO_2 insufflation and for an appropriate increase in pressure on the insufflator!

Now place the trocar for the scope in the skin incision 15 cm below the xiphoid and 1–2 fingers paramedian on the left. To do so use either

- a trocar with a sharp tip (10/12 mm) or
- a trocar with optical obturator.

When inserting the trocar, take care
- **to go in perpendicular to the abdominal wall,**
- **to support the trocar with the hand, and**
- **not to use excessive force in order to avoid blood vessel and organ injuries in the event of loss of resistance (→ p. 63, V-2; V-3)!**

PLACING THE WORKING TROCARS

Trocar for the scope T1 (10/12 mm) Working trocar T2 (5 mm or 10/12 mm; depending on the liver retracting device) Working trocar T3 (5 mm or 10/12 mm) Working trocar T4 (10/12 mm) Working trocar T5 (10/12 mm) Size 11 scalpel Reducer caps, if necessary

Insert the scope into the trocar (T1).

Then position the patient in a 30° reverse Trendelenburg position in order to make the small intestine slide into the lower abdomen by gravity and to obtain an optimal view of the operating field (→ p. 22, I).

Perform a diagnostic laparoscopy to make sure that there are no pathological changes and/or injuries which might require an alteration of the operative strategy or even prevent continuation of the operation (→ p. 63, V-2; V-3).

The liver is retracted through the trocar T2. The positions of the other working trocars depend on the operative site and are therefore established after the liver retracting device has been inserted.

Place the working trocar subcostally at the level of the xiphoid process. Choose the working trocar site T2 by palpating the abdominal wall under vision and use diaphanoscopy to ensure that no major cutaneous vessels will be injured when the trocar is inserted (→ p. 63, V-1; V-2).

T2: In the midline, subcostally at the level of the xiphoid process (depending on liver size and liver retracting device)

Incise the skin with a scalpel according to the trocar diameter: about 1 cm when using a 5 mm trocar and about 1.5 cm with a 10/12 mm trocar. Now insert the working trocar under direct vision.

Ensure that the skin incision is the right size!

When placing the trocar make sure that it points exactly towards the operating field, as later corrections will not be possible.

When placing the trocar, take care
- **to insert the trocar under direct vision to avoid injuries (→ p. 63, V-2; V-3), and**
- **to point the trocar exactly towards the operating field, as later corrections will be difficult, if not impossible in obese abdominal walls!**

After the liver retracting device has been inserted, an unrestricted view of the operating field should be guaranteed. Then fix the liver retracting device to the fixation arm.

Place the liver retracting device carefully and always under direct vision, as in obese patients the texture of the liver is often fat, which increases the vulnerability of the tissue (→ p. 64, V-3d)!

Choose the working trocar sites T3, T4 and T5 depending on the operative site, roughly in a half-moon around the trocar for the scope, and by palpating the abdominal wall under direct vision. Use diaphanoscopy to ensure that no major cutaneous vessels will be injured when the trocar is inserted (→ p. 63, V-1; V-2).

T3: In the left lateral abdomen
T4: In the right epigastrium, depending on liver size
T5: In the left epigastrium

Insert the trocars according to the above description for T2, starting with the skin incisions. Then insert the working trocars under direct vision.

When placing the trocars, take care
- **to insert the trocars under direct vision to avoid injuries (→ p. 63, V-2; V-3),**
- **to point the trocars exactly towards the operating field, as later corrections will be difficult, if not impossible in obese abdominal walls,**
- **to place additional trocars at any time to gain optimal working conditions, and**
- **to place the trocars with a minimum distance of 10 cm between them in order to avoid interference from scope and instruments!**

Remove the obturators from the trocars and attach the reducer caps to T3, T4 and T5, if necessary.

Alternative: If the liver is greatly enlarged, requiring the use of another liver retracting device, insert an additional trocar (T6). The location of the trocar depends on the intra-operative site.

There are many ways to position the trocars. We prefer the placement described above, but it should be the surgeon's choice!

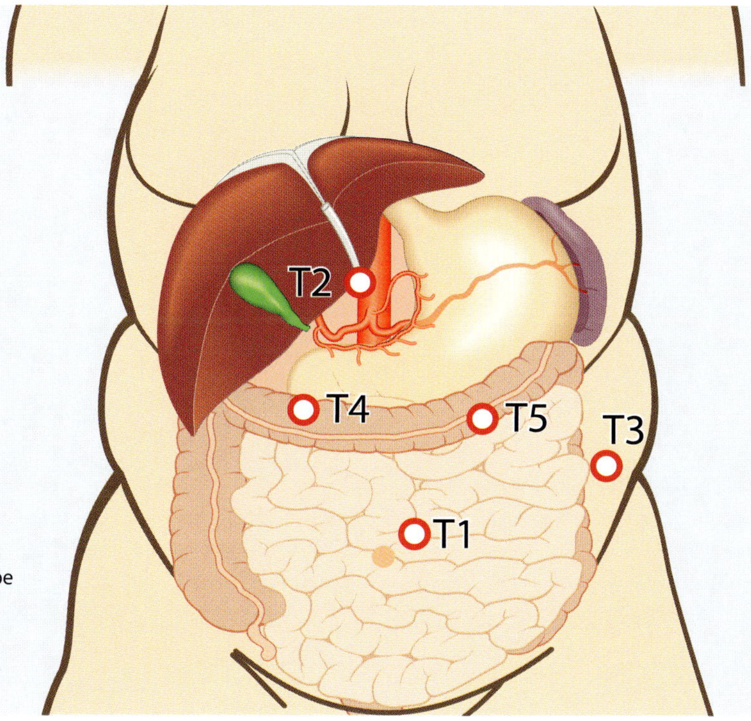

T1 Trocar for the scope
T2 Working trocar
T3 Working trocar
T4 Working trocar
T5 Working trocar

NODAL POINTS

01 Exploring the abdominal cavity

02 Identifying the anatomical landmarks

03 Creating the access to the bursa

04 Creating the gastric pouch

05 Dividing the omentum

06 Mobilizing the proximal jejunum

07 Creating the gastro-entero anastomosis

08 Closing the gastroenterostoma

09 Creating the entero-entero anastomosis

10 Closing the enterostoma

11 Dividing the intestine

12 Testing the gastro-entero anastomosis for leaks

13 Finishing the operation

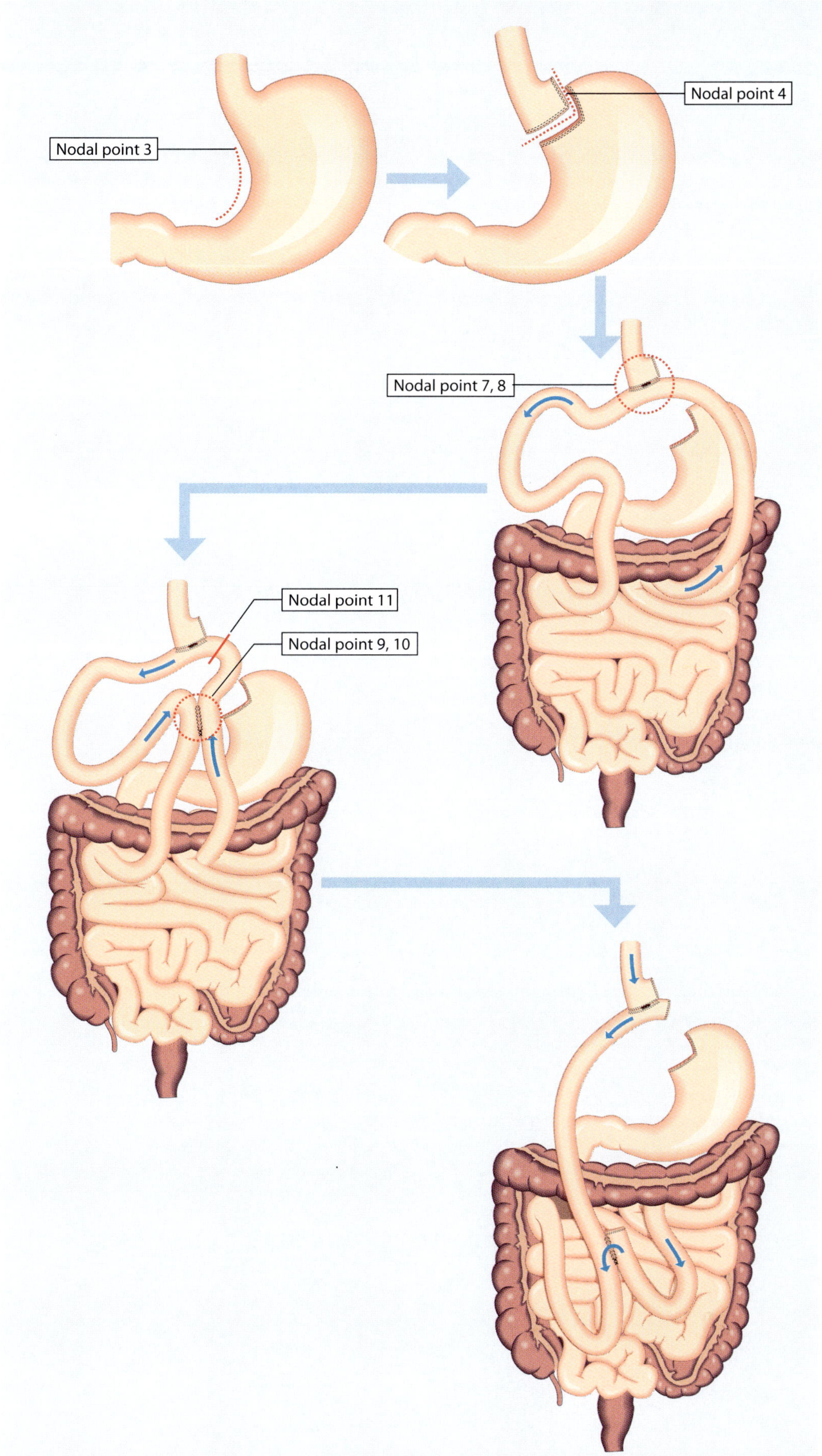
Nodal point 3
Nodal point 4
Nodal point 7, 8
Nodal point 11
Nodal point 9, 10

1 Exploring the abdominal cavity

T1	Scope
T2	Liver retracting device
T3	-
T4	Atraumatic grasping forceps, if necessary
T5	Harmonic® shears or curved scissors, if necessary

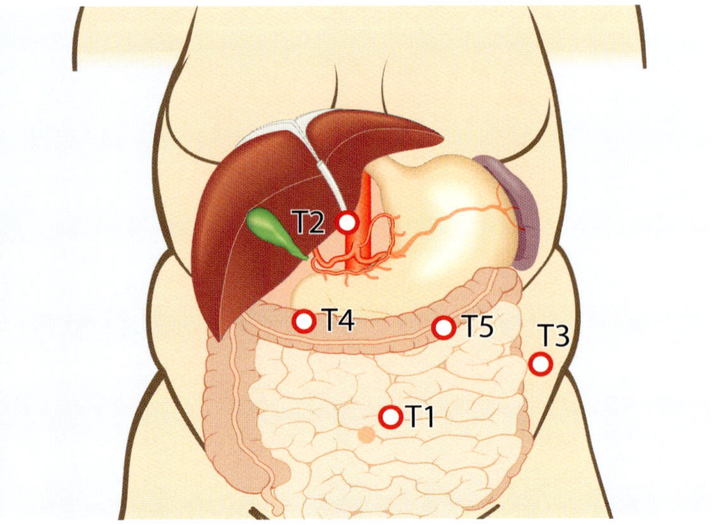

Examine the abdominal cavity carefully by inspecting it in a clockwise direction. Due to obesity a thorough inspection of the structures in the pelvis might be difficult.

- Pelvis: dome of the bladder, pouch of Douglas, the internal hernial orifices, and the uterus and adnexa in women
- Cecum with appendix
- Ascending colon
- Right upper abdomen: liver and gallbladder, right colonic flexure
- Greater omentum
- Transverse colon
- Left upper abdomen: stomach and spleen, splenic flexure
- Descending colon
- Sigmoid colon
- Jejunum and ileum

Look particularly for adhesions, erythema, vascular injections, serous fluid, pus, tumors and peritoneal carcinosis.

If a tumor or infection is found during the exploration, performing the gastric bypass is contraindicated!

Particularly check the trocar incision sites for adhesions and possible bleedings. Change the scope position, if necessary (→ p. 63, V-1; V-2).

Divide any adhesions in the operating field using sharp dissection (→ p. 63, V-1).

Divide any adhesions with organs promptly in order to avoid injuries (→ p. 63, V-3)!

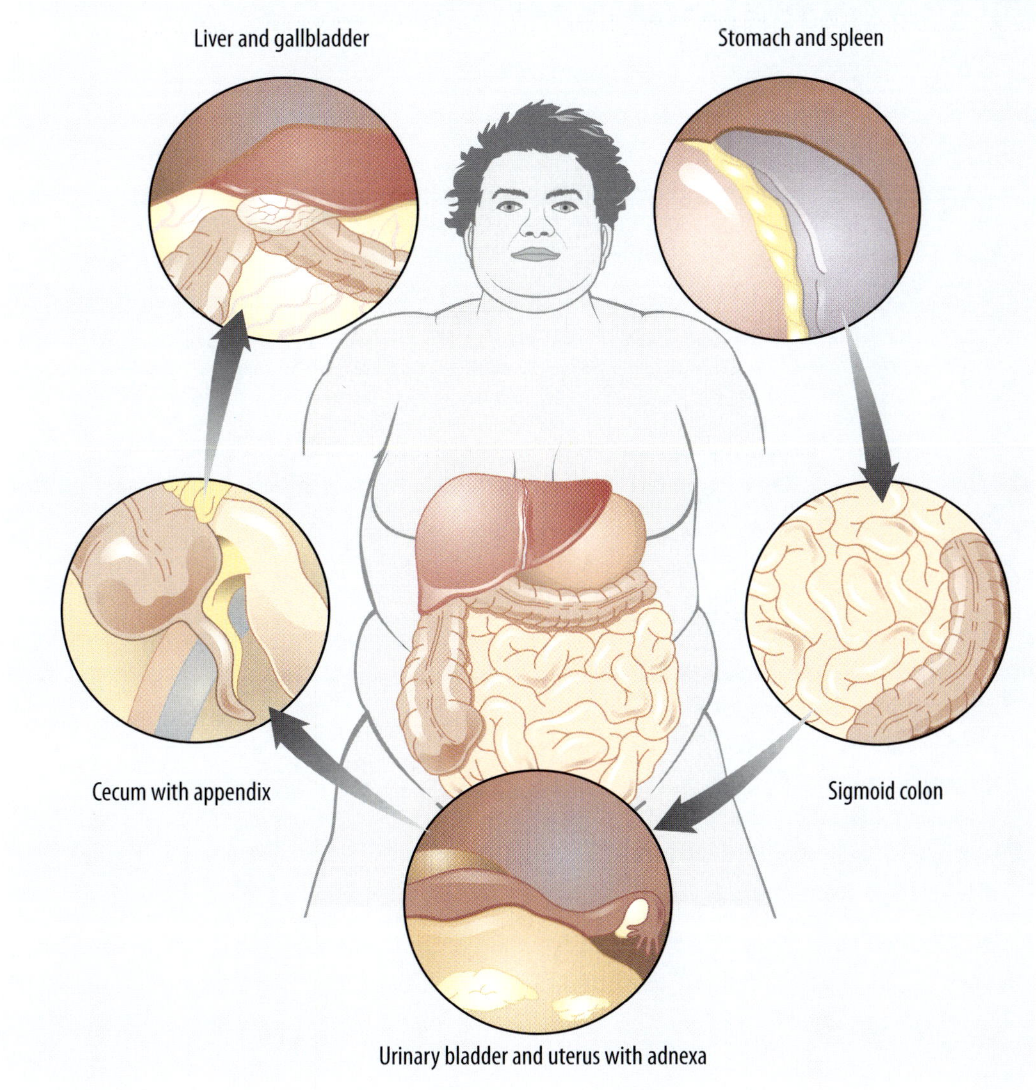
Liver and gallbladder
Stomach and spleen
Cecum with appendix
Sigmoid colon
Urinary bladder and uterus with adnexa

2 Identifying the anatomical landmarks

T1 Scope
T2 Liver retracting device
T3 -
T4 Atraumatic grasping forceps
T5 Harmonic® shears or curved scissors, if necessary

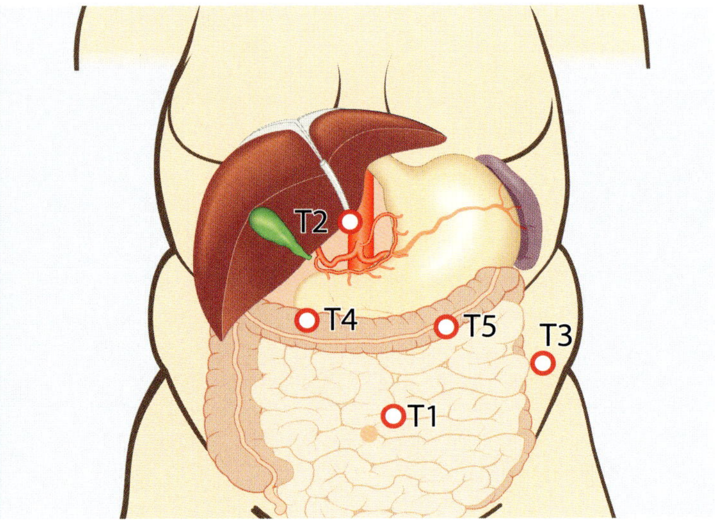

Identify the following anatomical landmarks:

Upper abdomen:

- Caudate and left liver lobe with falciform ligament
- Lesser omentum with hepatogastric ligament
- Left gastric artery, if possible
- Gastro-esophageal junction
- Stomach: lesser and greater curvature, angle of His
- Spleen with gastrophrenic ligament

In case of fat accumulations in the subcardiac region of the stomach and at the gastro-esophageal junction, use a dissector or sharp dissection to remove them in order to ensure an optimal view of the operating field.

Anatomical overview

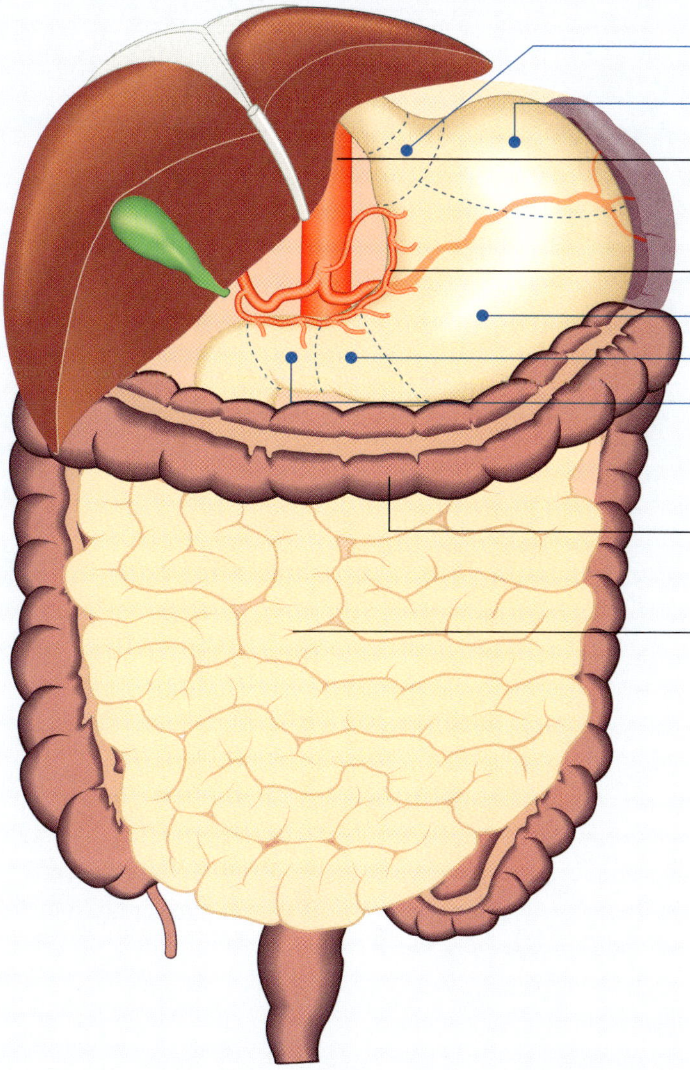

Overview of the operating field

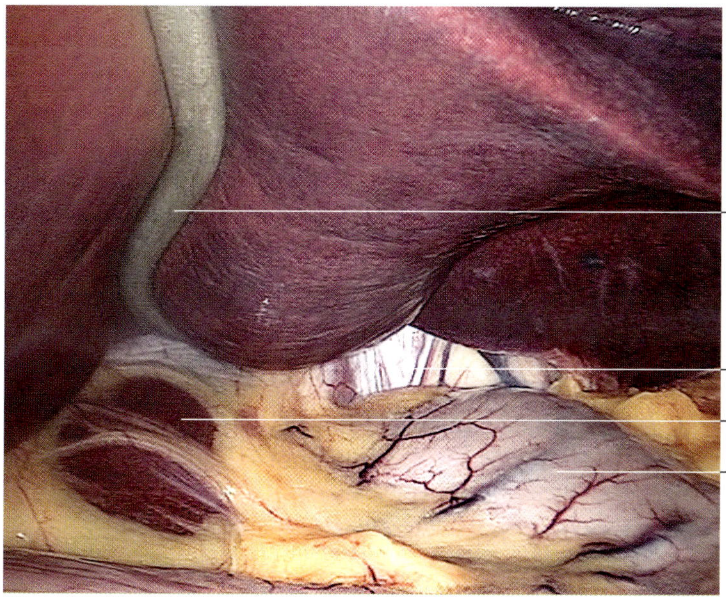

3 Creating the access to the bursa

T1 Scope
T2 Liver retracting device
T3 Atraumatic grasping forceps (assistant)
T4 Harmonic® shears
T5 Atraumatic grasping forceps

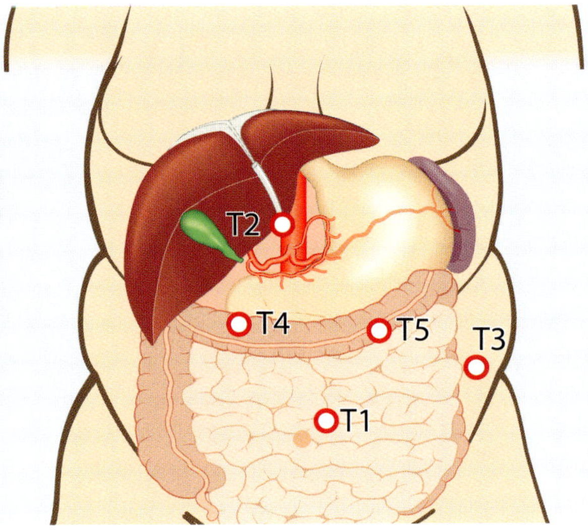

Grasp the fundus with an atraumatic forceps (T5) and pull it down to visualize the left crus of the diaphragm. Free the angle of His using the Harmonic® shears (T4) to reduce tension on the stomach.

Dissect the angle of His to reduce the tension on the stomach and to avoid injuries.

Have the assistant grasp the fundus and pull it laterally to the left (T3). Use the Harmonic® shears (T4) and open the omental bursa close to the lesser curvature approximately 4 cm distal to the cardia. Push the lesser curvature laterally and ventrally by using the atraumatic forceps (T5). Dissect the lesser curvature towards the gastro-esophageal junction. Take care not to injure the left gastric artery, as it assures the blood supply to the pouch (→ p. 63, V-2a).

Dissect close to the gastric wall and take care not to injure the left gastric artery as it assures the blood supply to the pouch.

Perform a retrogastric dissection by exploring the bursa. Use the Harmonic® shears (T4) and dissect layer for layer, carefully and under vision. Dissect in the direction of the left crus of the diaphragm.

Work under vision control to avoid any injuries to the gastric wall, spleen or other tissue.

Creating the access to the bursa

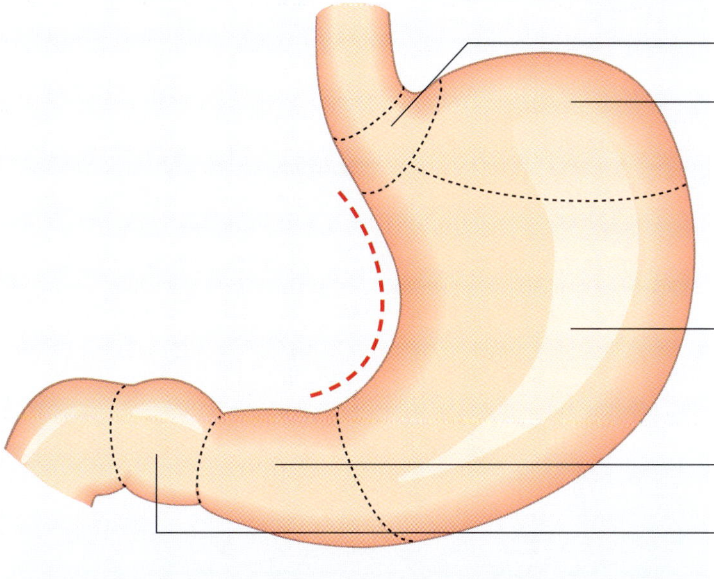

Opening the bursa

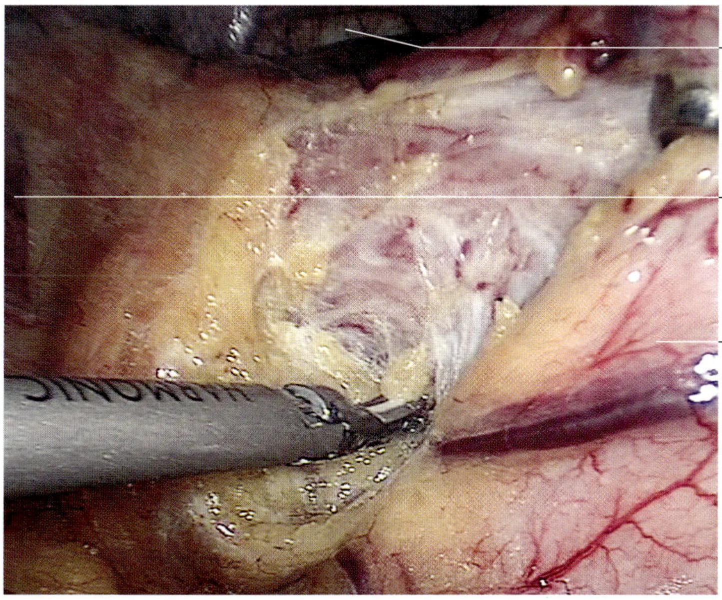

Access to the bursa

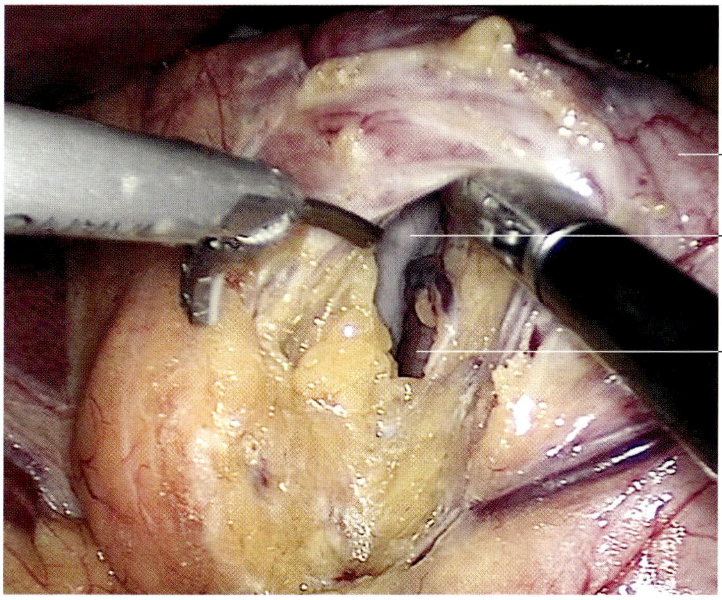

4 Creating the gastric pouch

T1 Scope
T2 Liver retracting device
T3 Atraumatic grasping forceps (assistant)
T4 Endoscopic linear cutter (45 mm cutter length), later atraumatic grasping forceps
T5 Atraumatic grasping forceps, later endoscopic linear cutter (45 mm cutter length)

– Different cartridges (depending on tissue thickness)

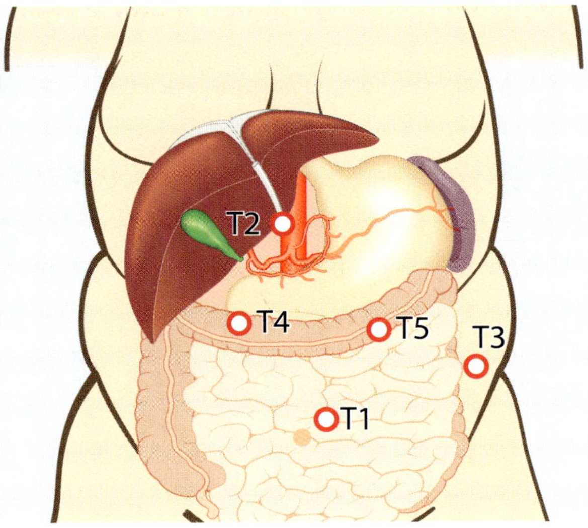

Use a gastric calibration tube with a balloon to ensure an optimal calibration of the pouch size.

Ask the anesthetist to pass the gastric calibration tube into the stomach and to slowly fill the balloon of the tube with 25 ml saline solution. Then tell him to draw the tube back into the cardia.

Note that the pouch size is less than 30 ml to ensure an adequate weight loss postoperatively.

Have the assistant insert an atraumatic forceps into the opened bursa behind the stomach (T3) to lift it ventrally.

Grasp the lesser curvature at the corpus with an atraumatic forceps (T5).

Insert the endoscopic linear cutter (T4) and place it horizontally below the cardia. Use gold or green cartridges (1.8/2.0 mm closed staple height) for the division of the stomach, depending on the thickness of the stomach wall.

Before closing the linear cutter be sure not to overtighten the stomach. This may cause an insufficient distance to the cardia.

Close the endoscopic linear cutter. In case of difficulty with closing the cutter, adjust the positioning of the jaws and grasp less tissue. An accumulation of tissue at the proximal end of the jaws may result in an incomplete staple line.

Take care not to accumulate tissue at the proximal jaws as this may result in an incomplete staple line.

Prior to firing, keep the endoscopic linear cutter closed for about 15 seconds. The accurate tissue compression minimizes the tissue liquid and ensures a proper staple formation and a safe staple line.

Fire the endoscopic linear cutter. Usually it is sufficient to create the horizontal staple line with 1 firing.

Then change instruments from T4 and T5 to perform the vertical staple line of the pouch.

Creating the gastric pouch

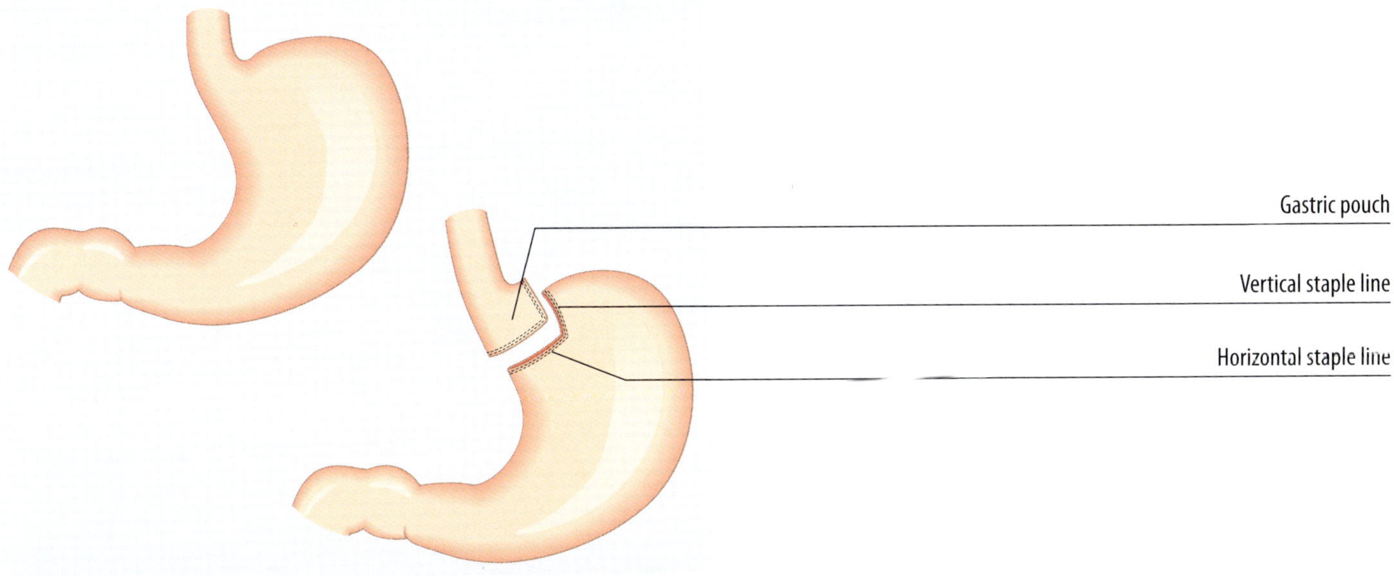

Placing the endoscopic linear cutter for horizontal staple line

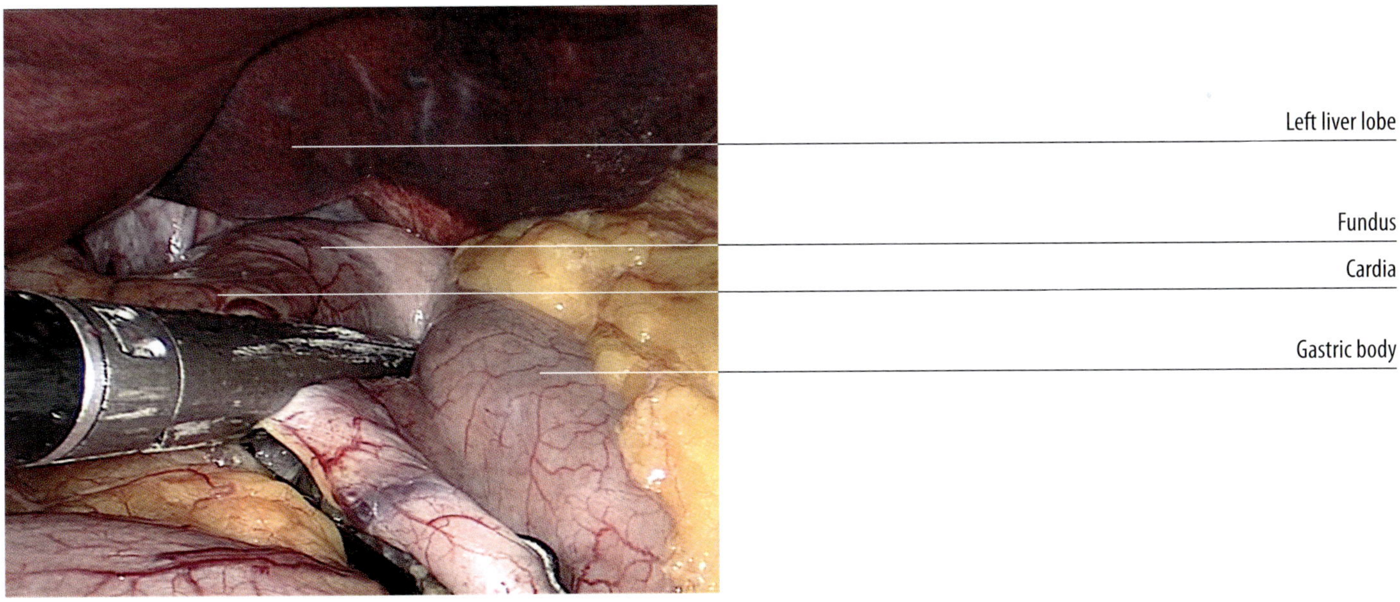

Horizontal staple line after firing

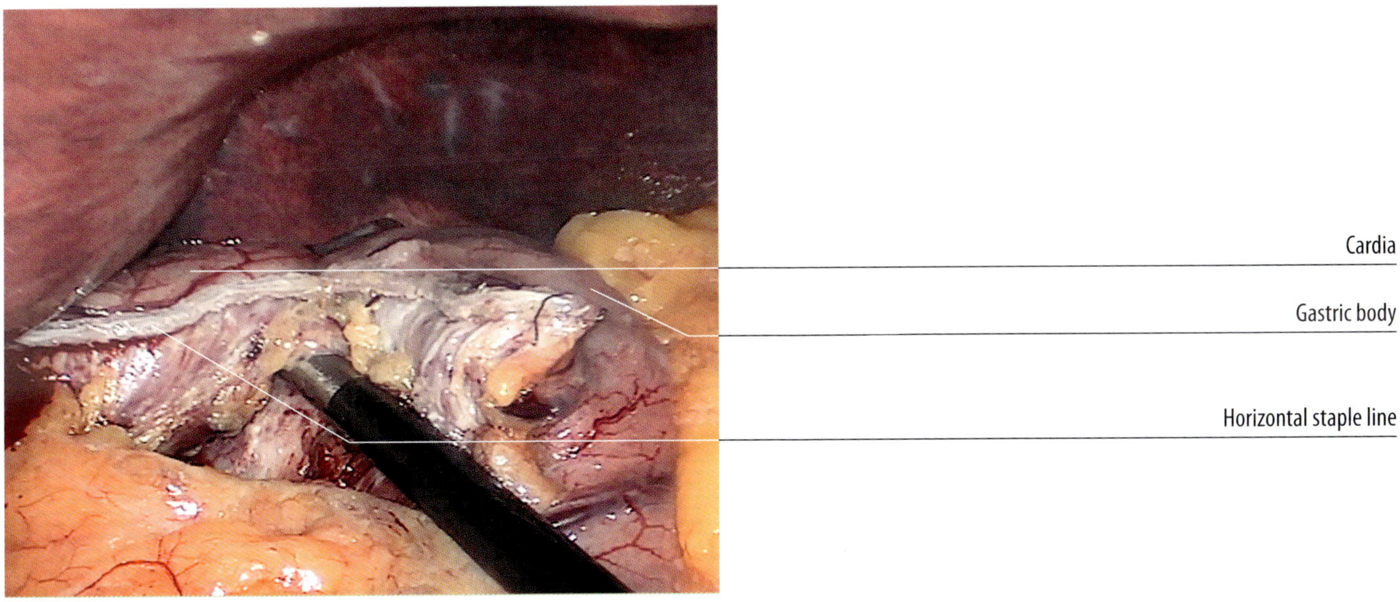

4 Creating the gastric pouch

T1 Scope
T2 Liver retracting device
T3 Atraumatic grasping forceps (assistant)
T4 Atraumatic grasping forceps
T5 Endoscopic linear cutter (45 mm cutter length)

– Different cartridges (depending on tissue thickness)

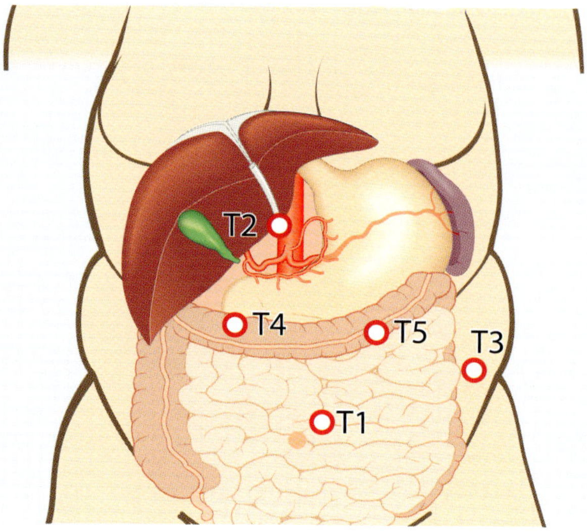

Grasp the proximal stomach with an atraumatic forceps (T4) and pull it laterally to the right.

Have the assistant push the opened bursa laterally to the left by using an atraumatic forceps (T3).

Then place the endoscopic linear cutter (T5) at the left lateral end of the staple line in a vertical direction up to the angle of His. Use the left crus of the diaphragm as the landmark for the division.

Close and fire the endoscopic linear cutter as described above. Re-do the firings until the angle of His is reached and the pouch is created. Usually it is sufficient to create the vertical staple line with 1–2 firings. The need of 4 cartridges indicates that the pouch is too big.

Staple in a linear fashion.

Take care to staple in a linear fashion to avoid sacculations which may lead to dilatation or insufficiency.

Transect the stomach completely.

Take care to transect the stomach completely to avoid the development of gastro-gastric fistula postoperatively (→ p. 87, appendices).

Note that staple line bleeding is not unusual (→ p. 63, V-3c).

Alternative: Using buttress material may reduce the risk of staple line bleeding.

Dividing the stomach

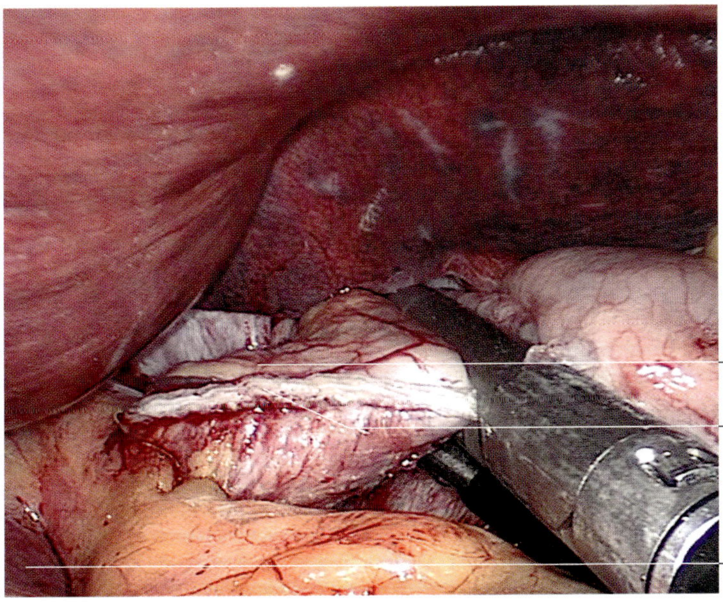

Second firing of vertical staple line

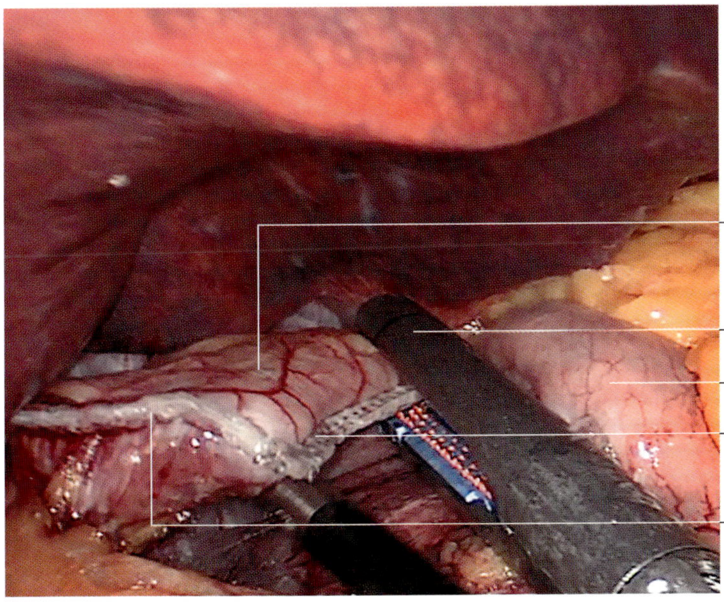

5 Dividing the omentum

T1 Scope
T2 Liver retracting device
T3 Atraumatic grasping forceps (assistant)
T4 Atraumatic grasping forceps
T5 Harmonic® shears

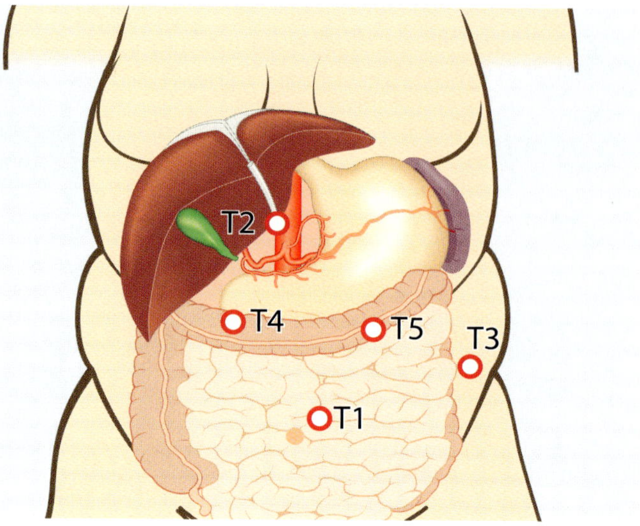

Dividing the greater omentum simplifies the mobilization of the proximal jejunum.

Have the assistant grasp the greater omentum with an atraumatic forceps (T3) and pull it laterally to the left.

Grasp the greater omentum with a second atraumatic forceps (T4), pull it laterally to the right.

Divide the omentum in cranial direction using the Harmonic® shears (T5), aiming from the level of T5 towards the pouch. Divide the omentum up to the transverse colon and leave the gastrocolic ligament intact. Take care not to injure the blood-supplying vessels of the colon (→ p. 63, V-2, V-3).

Take care not to injure the colon's blood-supplying vessels or the gastro-epiploic artery while dividing the omentum.

Dividing the omentum

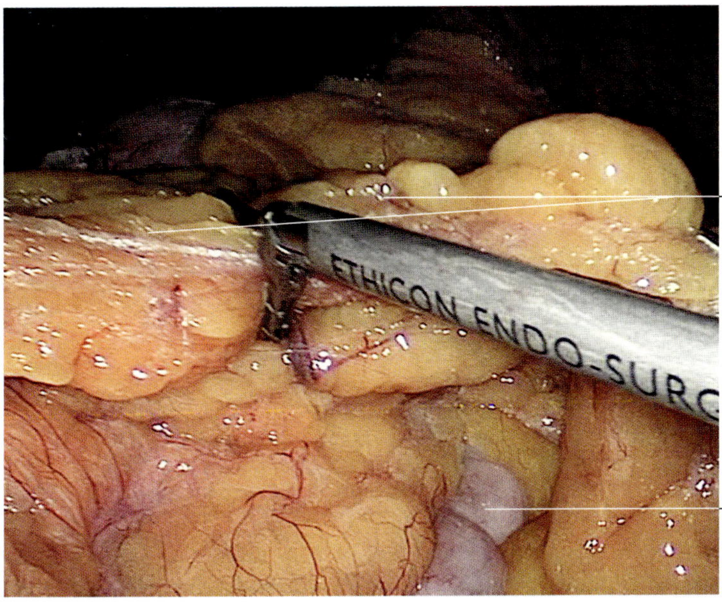

Dividing the omentum up to the transverse colon

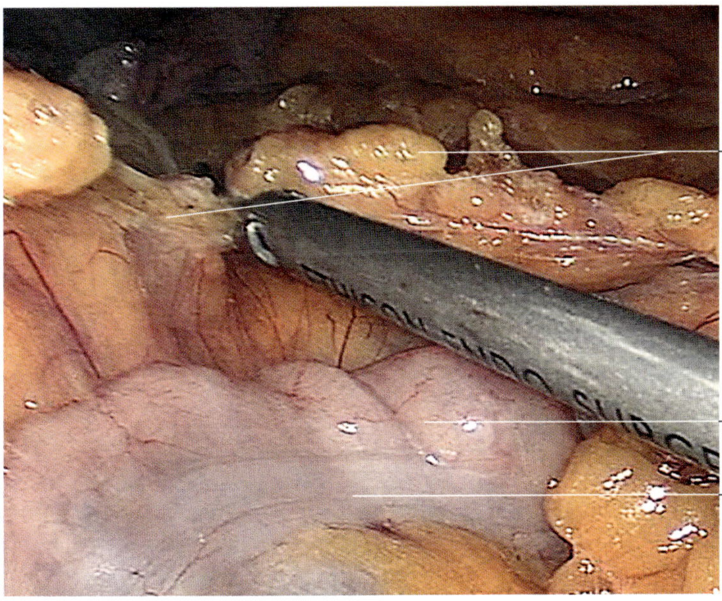

6 Mobilizing the proximal jejunum

T1 Scope
T2 Liver retracting device
T3 Atraumatic grasping forceps (assistant)
T4 Atraumatic grasping forceps
T5 Atraumatic grasping forceps with landmark

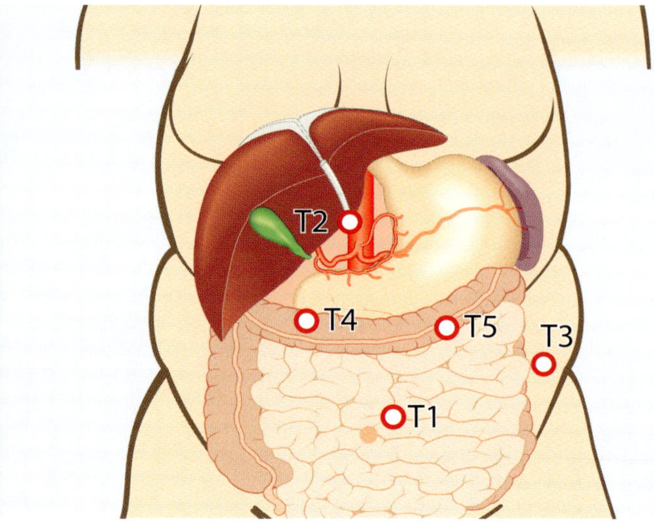

Have the assistant grasp the transverse colon with an atraumatic forceps through T3 and lift it up.

Identify the ligament of Treitz.

Grasp the intestine at the ligament of Treitz with an atraumatic forceps (T4) and place it to the patient´s left side by twisting the intestine 180° in a clockwise direction. The downstream-running intestinal part will thus be on the patient's right side.

Grasp the intestine (T5) step by step downstream and measure a distance to the ligament of Treitz of 20–50 cm. The length of this future bilio-pancreatic limb is a subject of controversy. In any case, it should be long enough to reach up to the gastric pouch.

Identifying the ligament of Treitz is obligatory to avoid a mix-up of the intestinal upstream/downstream orientation (→ p. 87, appendices).

Pay attention to work under strict vision control in order to minimize the risk of – often unrecognized – intestinal perforations, as they are one of the insidious complications (→ p. 64, V-3f).

Alternative: Placing a marker clip on the selected intestinal part helps to avoid a mix-up of the intestinal upstream/downstream orientation, which could have fatal consequences.

Identifying the ligament of Treitz

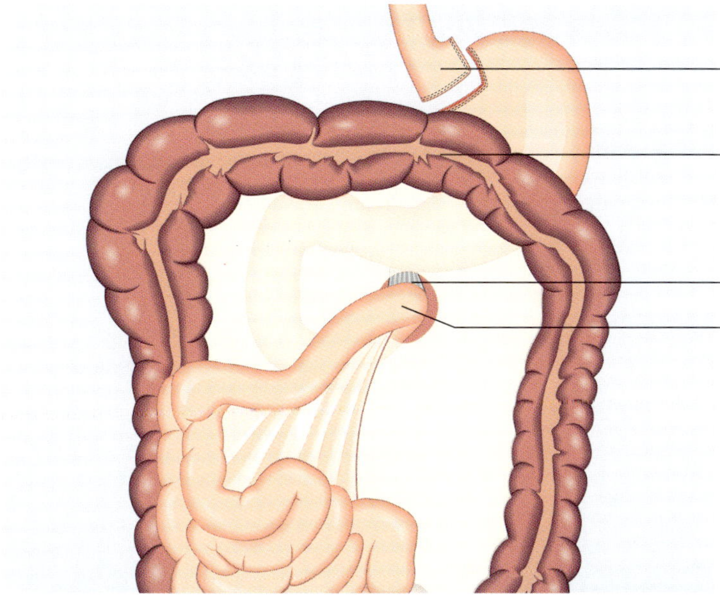

Measuring the intestine

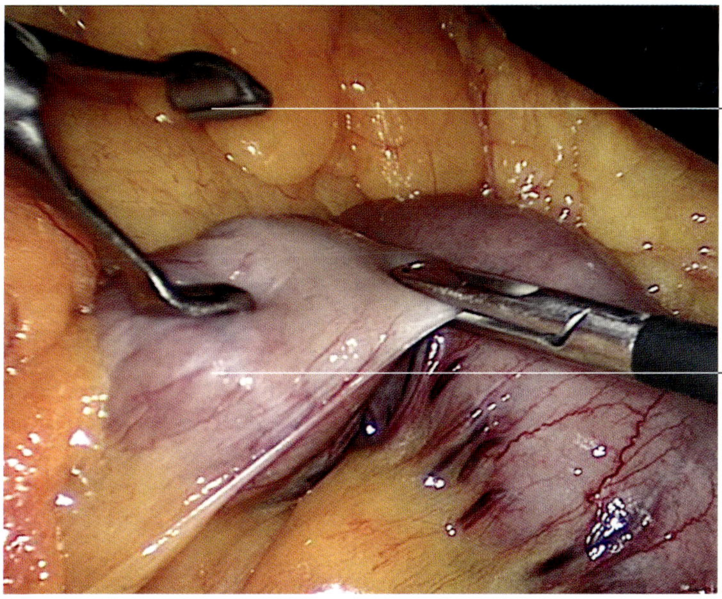

7 Creating the gastro-entero anastomosis

T1 Scope
T2 Liver retracting device
T3 Atraumatic grasping forceps (assistant)
T4 Atraumatic grasping forceps
T5 Harmonic® shears, later sharp scissors, later endoscopic linear cutter

– Different cartridges (depending on tissue thickness)

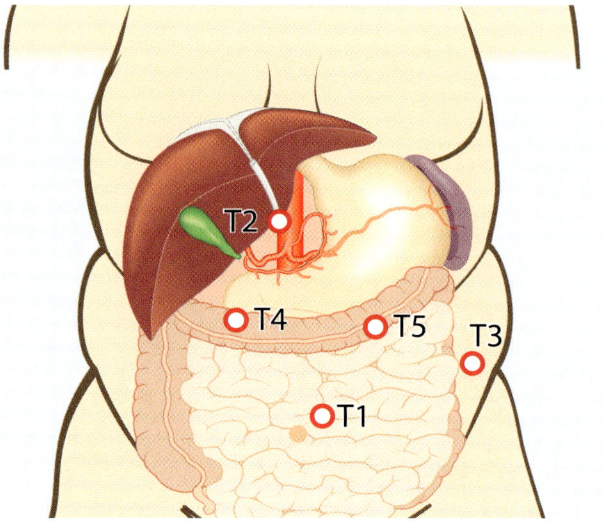

Use the Harmonic® shears (T5) and perform a small enterotomy in the measured intestinal region (20–50 cm from the ligament of Treitz).

Grasp the pouch with an atraumatic forceps (T4) and perform a gastrotomy through the horizontal staple line using sharp scissors (T5). Since the mucosa of the pouch will be trapped in the staple line, this is the easiest way to gain access to the lumen.

Avoid a blunt dissection of the pouch which may create a lumen in the submucosal space, thus preventing proper access to the pouch.

Grasp the intestine with an atraumatic forceps (T4). Insert the endoscopic linear cutter (T5) with a blue or gold cartridge (1.5/1.8 mm closed staple height), depending on the thickness of the stomach wall and intestinal wall. Introduce the anvil into the opening of the intestine in an upstream direction.

Place the intestine with the endoscopic linear cutter (T5) in front of the pouch. Grasp the right side of the pouch with an atraumatic forceps (T4). Have the assistant grasp the left side of the pouch with an atraumatic forceps (T3).

Be sure that the future bilio-pancreatic limb is on the patient´s left side and that the future alimentary limb is on the patient's right side.

Place the stapler cartridge into the opening of the pouch to connect the intestine to the pouch. Avoid excessive pushing of the cutter when connecting the intestine to the pouch.

Avoid excessive pushing of the cutter when connecting the intestine to the pouch. This could cause perforation of the intestine distal to the anastomosis (→ p. 64, V-3f).

Close the endoscopic linear cutter. Prior to firing, keep the linear cutter closed for about 15 seconds. The accurate tissue compression minimizes the tissue liquid and ensures proper and safe stapling.

Fire the endoscopic linear cutter.

Open the jaws of the linear cutter and remove the instrument.

Creating the gastro-entero anastomosis

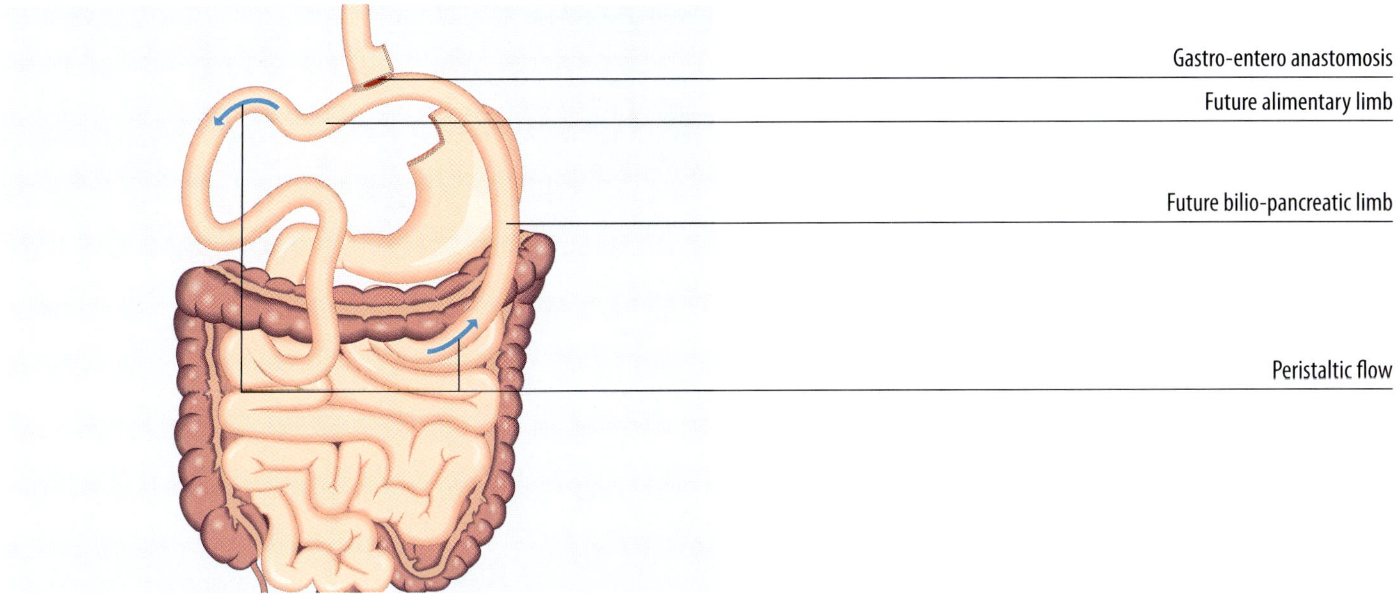

Opening the pouch with sharp scissors

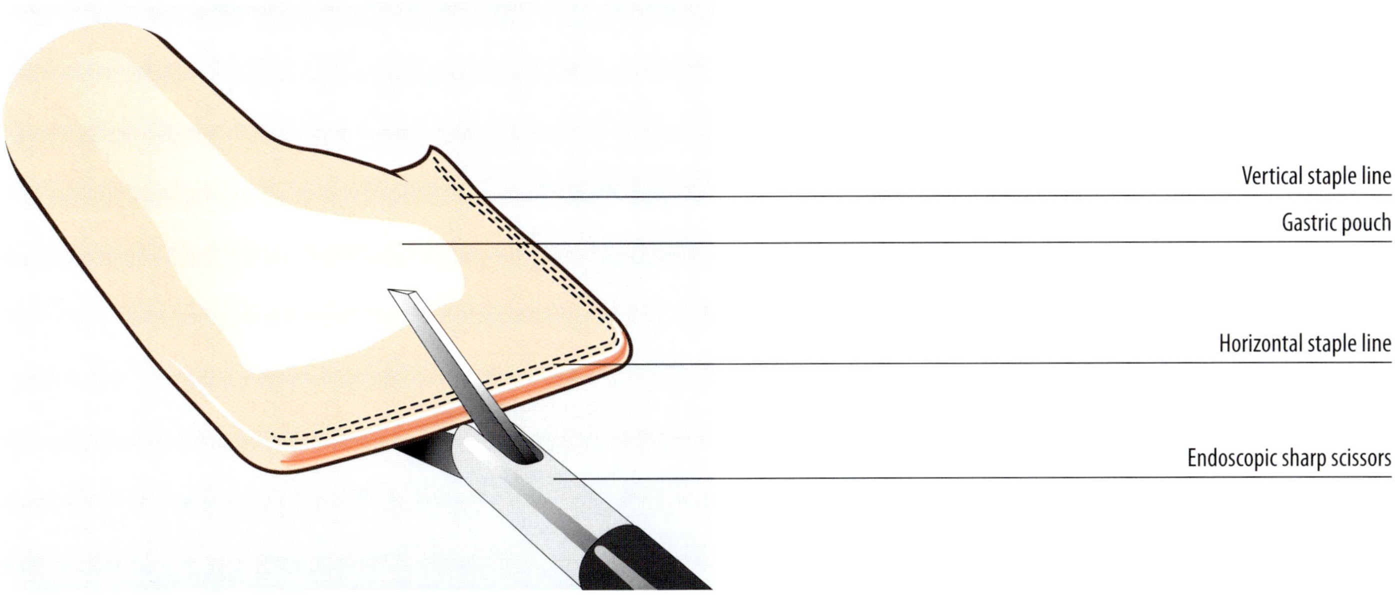

Connecting the intestine to the pouch

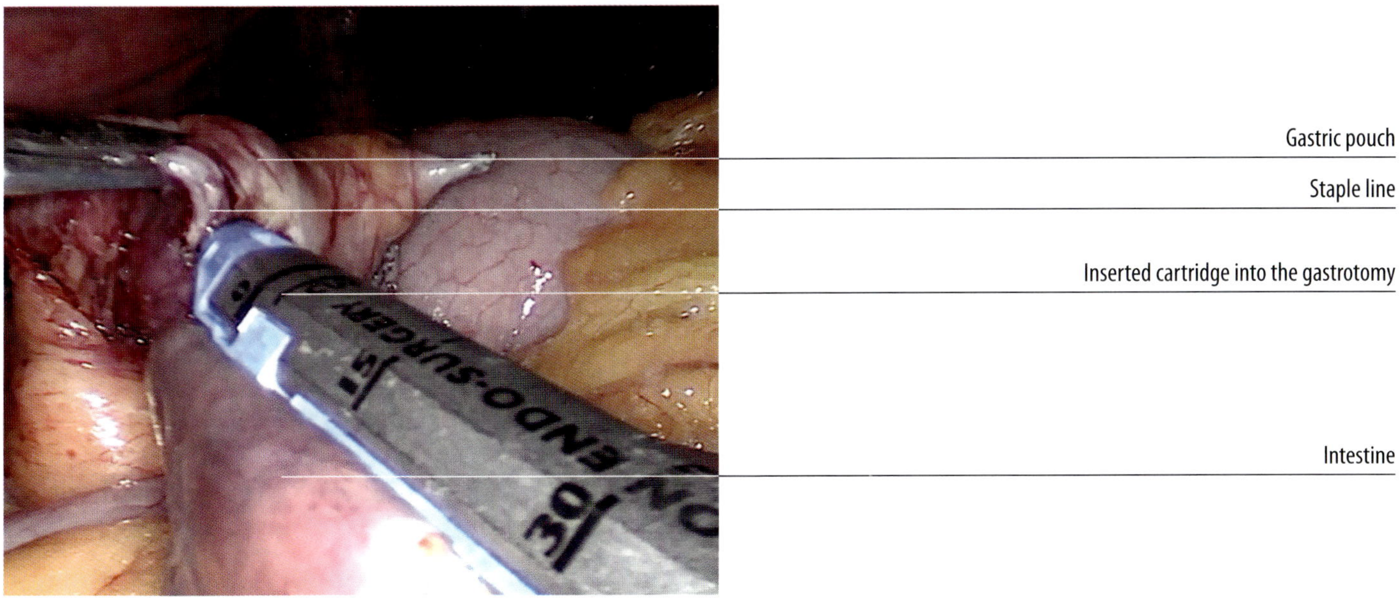

8 Closing the gastroenterostoma

T1 Scope
T2 Liver retracting device
T3 –
T4 Atraumatic grasping forceps
T5 Needle holder, later suture clip applier

- Absorbable sutures 3–0 (e.g. Vicryl™)
- Absorbable suture clips (e.g. LAPRA-TY®)

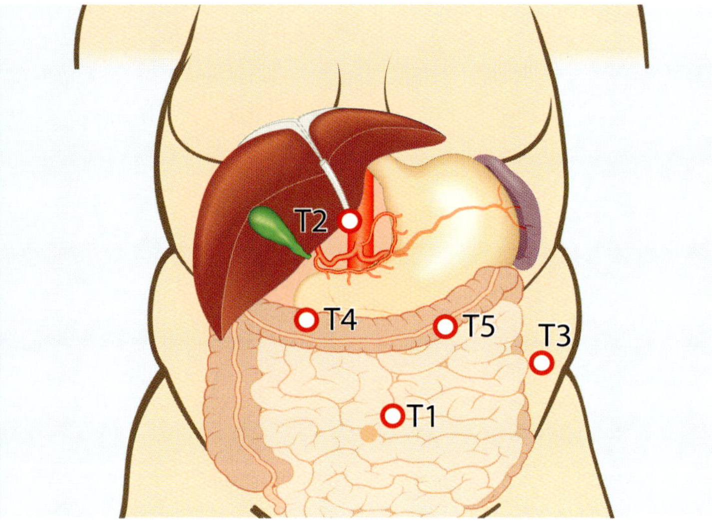

Grasp the intestine with an atraumatic forceps (T4). Insert a needle holder with a 3–0 absorbable suture (T5) and place an interrupted suture on the right lateral end of the remaining opening. Place seromuscular stitches on the intestinal side, but full thickness stitches through the stomach wall.

Always place seromuscular stitches through the intestinal wall but full thickness stitches through the stomach wall. This achieves a proper hemostasis of the pouch wall.

Insert another 3–0 absorbable suture (T5) and close the opening with a single-layer running suture from the left lateral side to the right. Place an absorbable suture clip using a clip applier to fix the suture.

Alternative: Using absorbable sutures with final knots instead of absorbable suture clips is also feasible. Using absorbable suture clips provides the advantage of a re-adjustable suture which ensures a proper size and forming of the closing.

Closing the gastroenterostoma

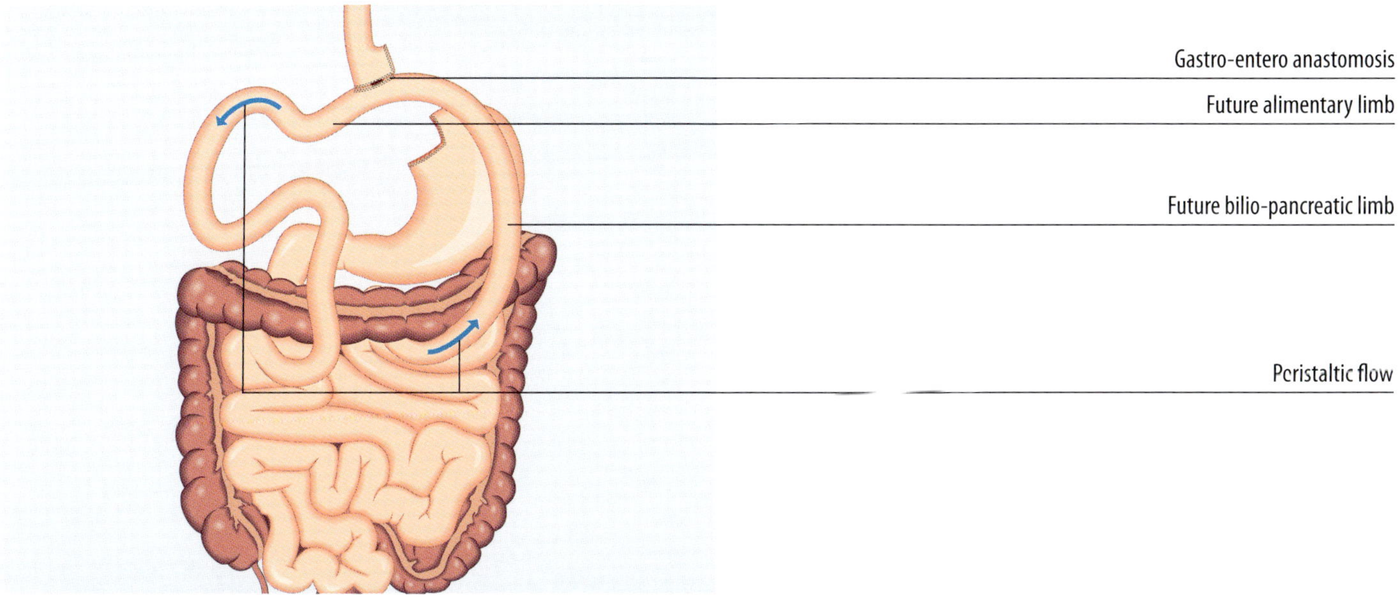

Suturing the gastro-entero anastomosis

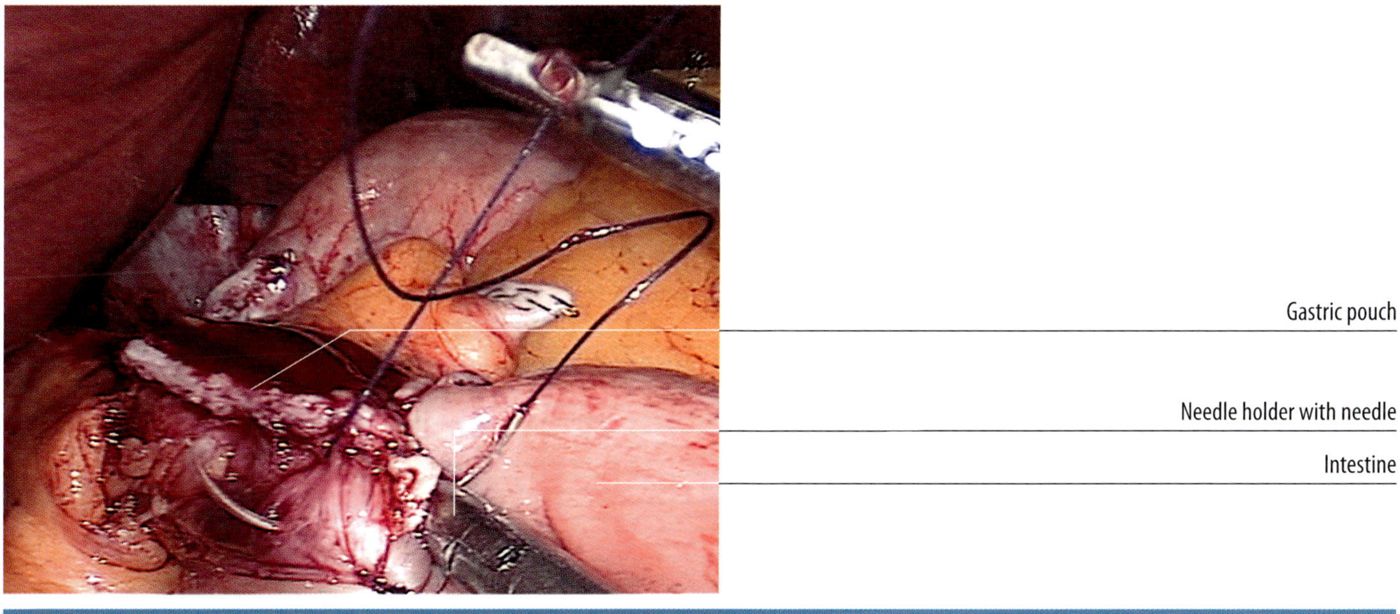

Placing an absorbable clip

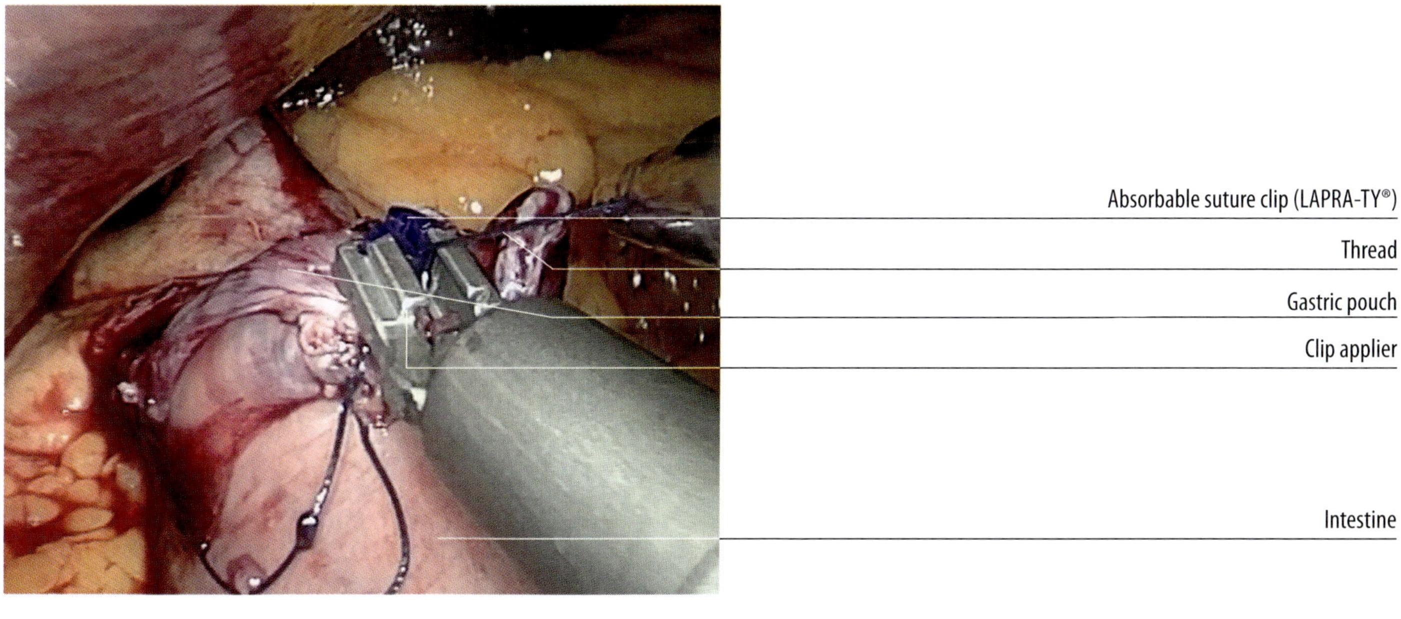

9 Creating the entero-entero anastomosis

- T1 Scope
- T2 Liver retracting device
- T3 Atraumatic grasping forceps (assistant)
- T4 Atraumatic grasping forceps
- T5 Atraumatic forceps with landmark, later Harmonic® shears, later endoscopic linear cutter

– Different cartridges (depending on tissue thickness)

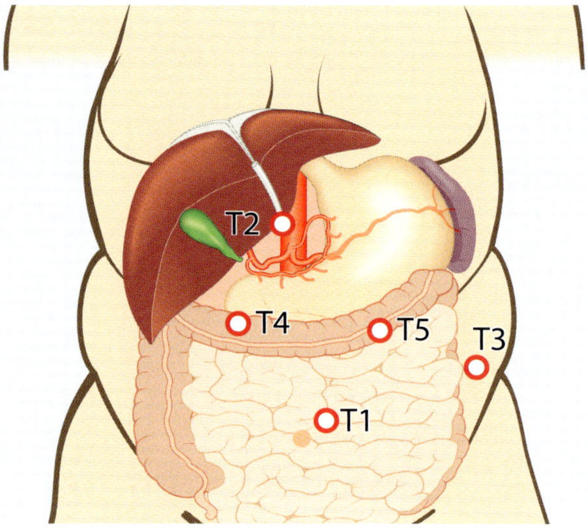

Grasp the intestine with atraumatic forceps (T4 and T5) at the gastro-entero anastomosis and measure step by step a distance of 120–150 cm from the gastro-entero anastomosis in downstream direction. There is a lack of consensus and no hard evidence for deciding on the length of the alimentary limb. The authors usually prefer a length of 120 cm.

Remove the atraumatic forceps from T5 and insert it through T3. Have the assistant grasp the intestine with the atraumatic forceps (T3). Perform an enterotomy in the measured intestine using the Harmonic® shears (T5).

Grasp the future bilio-pancreatic limb near to the gastro-entero anastomosis with an atraumatic forceps (T4) and perform an enterotomy in a distance of 3–5 cm to the gastro-entero anastomosis using the Harmonic® shears (T5).

Place the enterotomy of the future alimentary limb beside the enterotomy of the future bilio-pancreatic limb. Take care that the two limbs have antiparallel upstream/downstream orientation.

Take care that the two limbs have antiparallel upstream/downstream orientation (→ p. 87, appendices).

Insert the endoscopic linear cutter (T5) loaded with white or blue cartridges (1.0/1.5 mm closed staple height), depending on the thickness of the intestinal wall.

To create a side to side anastomosis, place the stapler anvil into the opening of the future alimentary limb in an upstream direction and place the stapler cartridge into the future bilio-pancreatic limb in a downstream direction.

Close the endoscopic linear cutter.

Prior to firing, keep the linear cutter closed for about 15 seconds. Accurate tissue compression minimizes the tissue liquid and ensures proper and safe stapling.

Fire the endoscopic linear cutter. Open the jaws of the endoscopic linear cutter.

Perform a second firing with the endoscopic linear cutter in downstream direction to ensure a sufficient diameter of the entero-entero anastomosis.

Alternative: Placing a marker clip on the selected intestinal part helps to avoid a mix-up of the intestinal upstream/downstream orientation, which could have fatal consequences.

Creating the entero-entero anastomosis

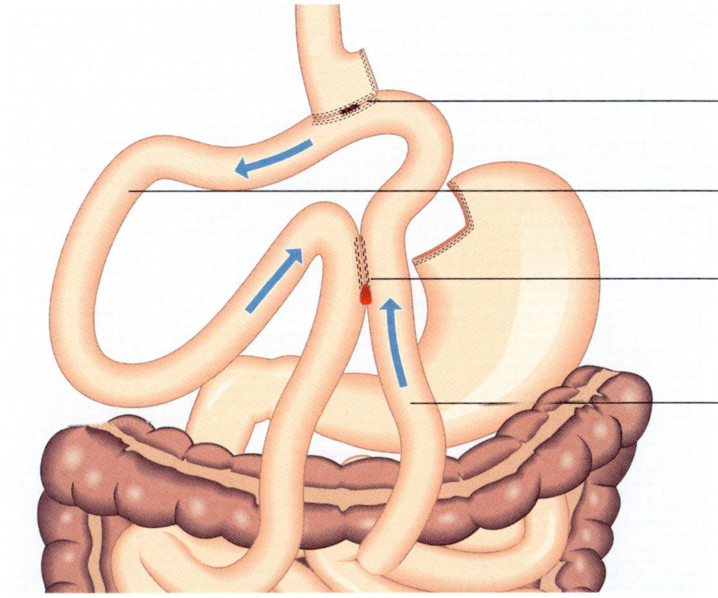

Enterotomy in a distance of 120 cm to the gastro-entero anastomosis

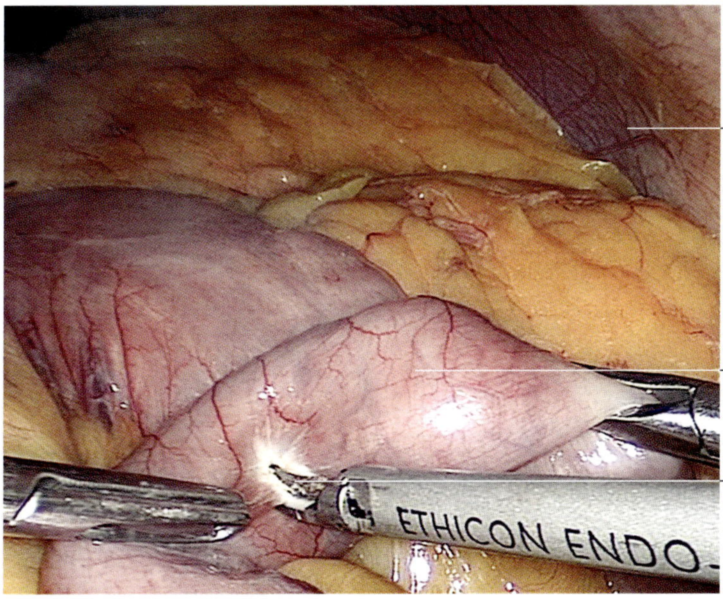

Stapling with the endoscopic linear cutter

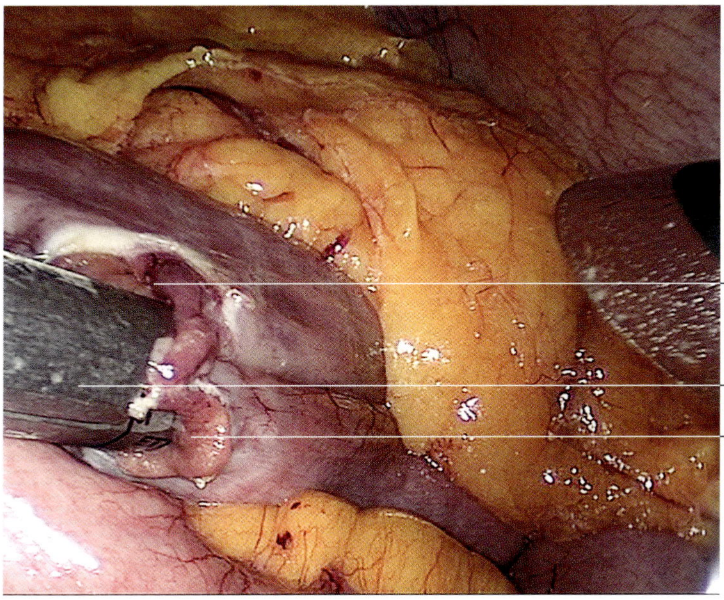

10 Closing the enterostoma

T1 Scope
T2 Liver retracting device
T3 Atraumatic grasping forceps (assistant)
T4 Atraumatic grasping forceps
T5 Needle holder, later suture clip applier

- Absorbable sutures 3–0 (e.g. Vicryl™)
- Absorbable suture clips (e.g. LAPRA-TY®)

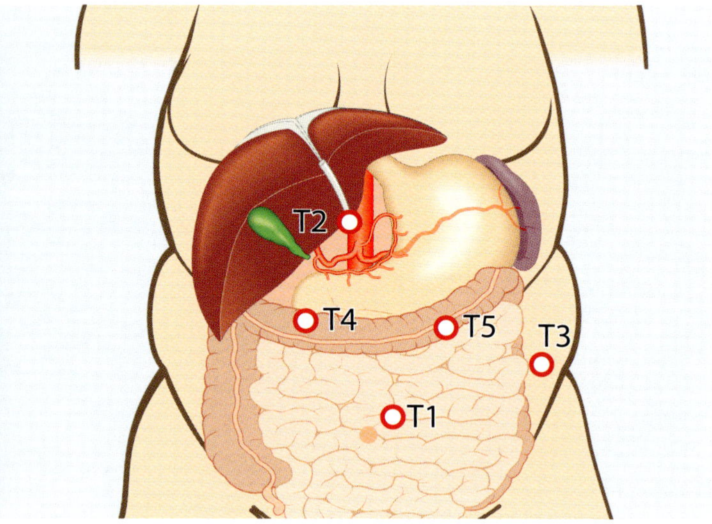

Grasp the alimentary limb with an atraumatic forceps (T4).

Insert a needle holder with a 3–0 absorbable thread (T5) and place an interrupted suture at the distal end of the opening. Do not cut the end of the thread. Have the assistant grasp the thread and pull it caudally.

Insert another 3–0 absorbable thread and place a single layer running suture, starting at the proximal end and running downwards in a longitudinal direction. Do not cut the beginning of this thread. Ask the assistant to grasp that thread and to pull it cranially (T3). Perform the running suture with seromuscular stitches.

Avoid excessive suturing as this may narrow the entero-entero anastomosis or even the alimentary limb. This could cause high intestinal obstruction with a risk of dilation of the remnant stomach. This complication can be fatal (→ p. 87, appendices)!

Place an absorbable suture clip to close the suture.

Alternative: Using absorbable sutures with final knots instead of absorbable suture clips is also feasible. Using absorbable suture clips provides the advantage of a re-adjustable suture, which ensures a proper size and forming of the closing.

Closing the enterostoma

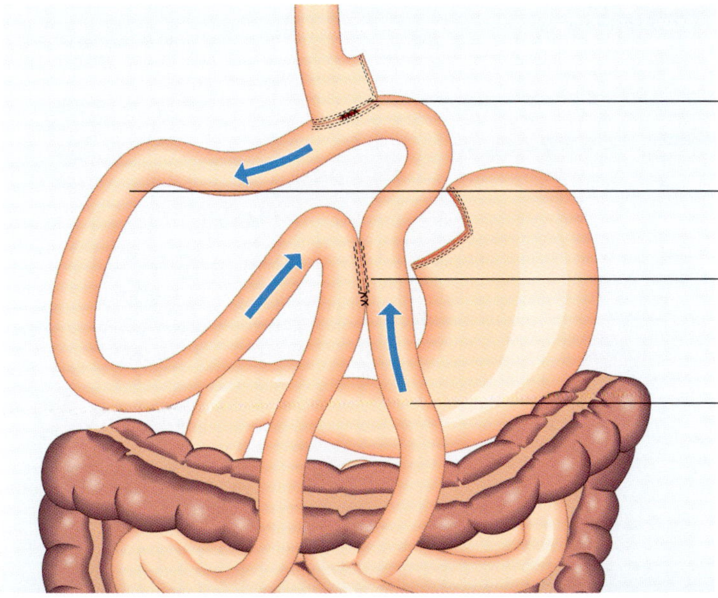

Suturing the entero-entero anastomosis

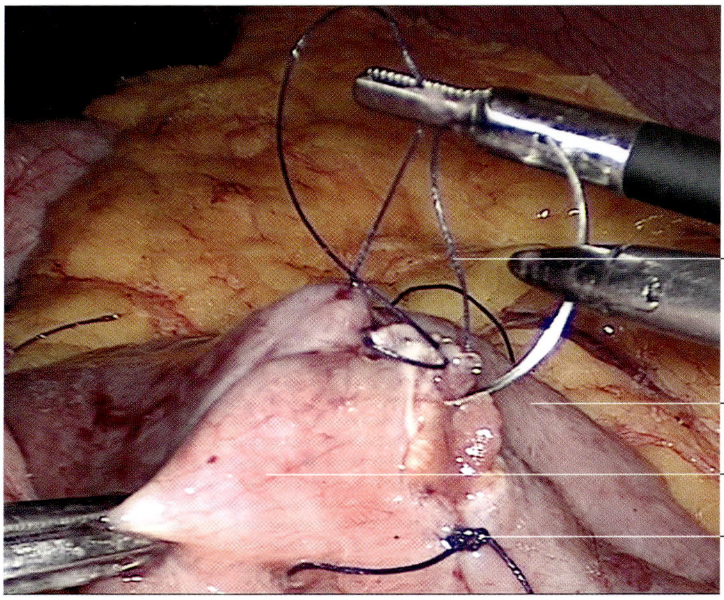

LAPRA-TY® fixed running suture

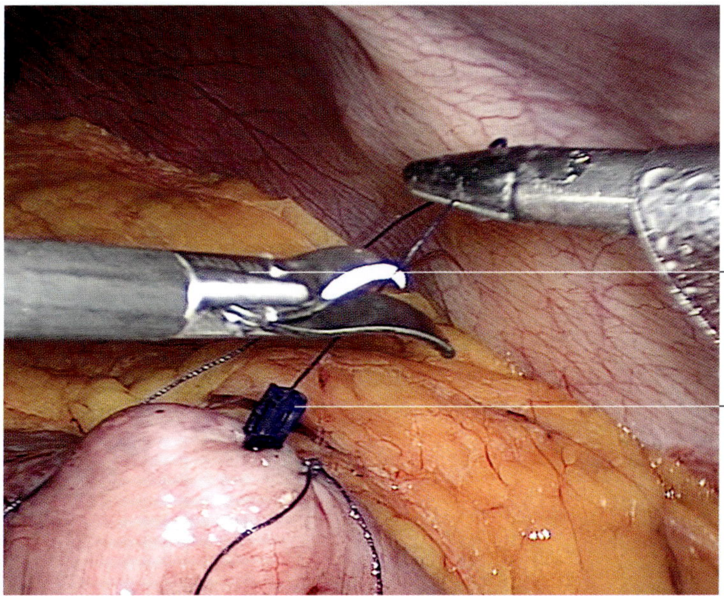

11 Dividing the intestine

T1 Scope
T2 Liver retracting device
T3 Atraumatic grasping forceps (assistant)
T4 Harmonic® shears, later endoscopic linear cutter
T5 Atraumatic grasping forceps

– Different cartridges (depending on tissue thickness)

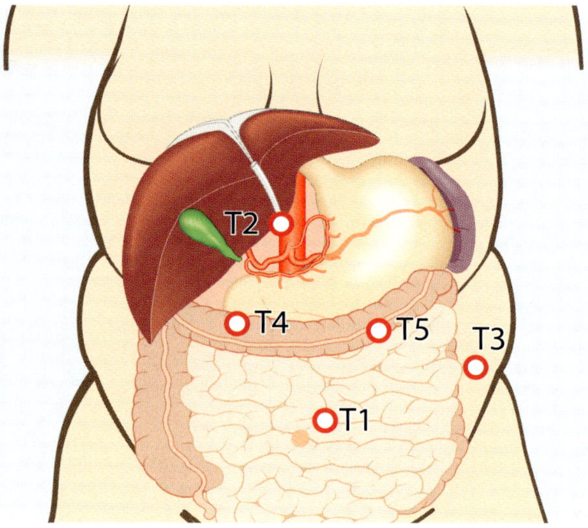

Ask the assistant to grasp the intestine between the gastro-entero and the entero-entero anastomosis with an atraumatic forceps (T3) and lift it up.

Slip the mesentery dorsally, using an atraumatic forceps through T5.

Perform a small opening through the intestinal mesentery between the gastro-entero and the entero-entero anastomosis close to the intestinal wall using the Harmonic® shears (T4).

Insert the endoscopic linear cutter (T4) loaded with white or blue cartridges (1.0/1.5 mm closed staple height), depending on the thickness of the intestinal wall. Place the anvil into the opening of the mesentery.

Divide the intestine near to the pouch to minimize the risk of an intestinal blind end at the gastro-entero anastomosis.

To avoid an intestinal blind end at the gastro-entero anastomosis, take care to divide the intestine near to the pouch.

Close the endoscopic linear cutter and keep the trigger closed for 15 seconds.

Fire the endoscopic linear cutter. Open the jaws and remove the linear cutter.

Note: By dividing the intestine between the gastro-entero anastomosis and the entero-entero anastomosis an antecolic antegastric alimentary limb is performed.

Staple line

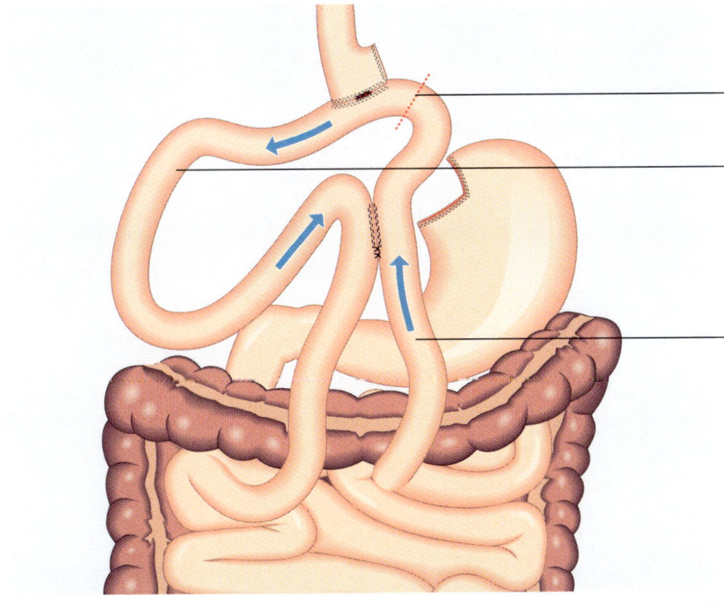

Dividing the intestine between gastro-entero and entero-entero anastomosis

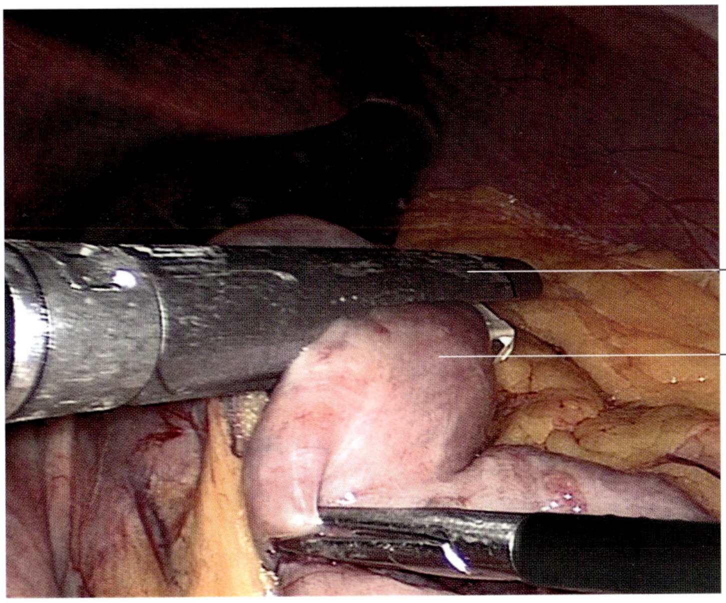

Created gastric bypass

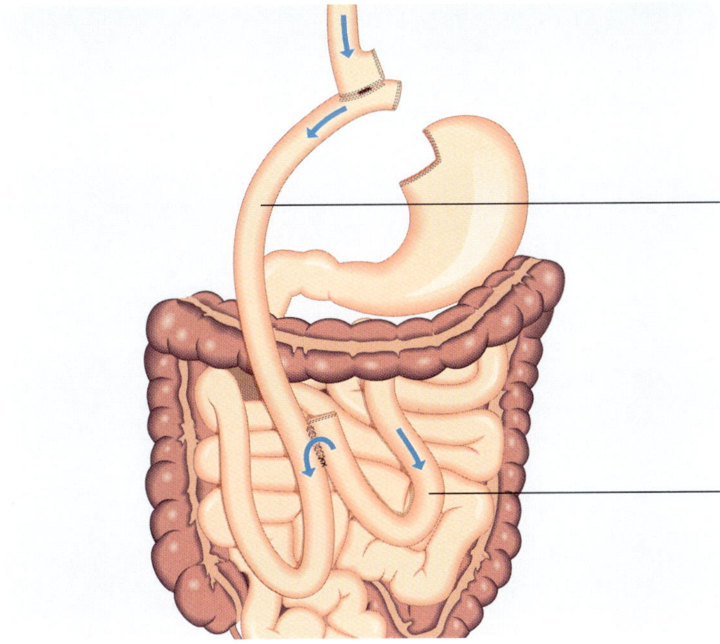

12 Testing the gastro-entero anastomosis for leaks

T1 Scope
T2 Liver retracting device
T3 –
T4 Atraumatic grasping forceps
T5 Atraumatic grasping forceps

- Bowl with 20 ml methylene blue solution (5 ml methylene blue 1 % with 15 ml saline solution)
- 10 ml syringe with methylene blue solution

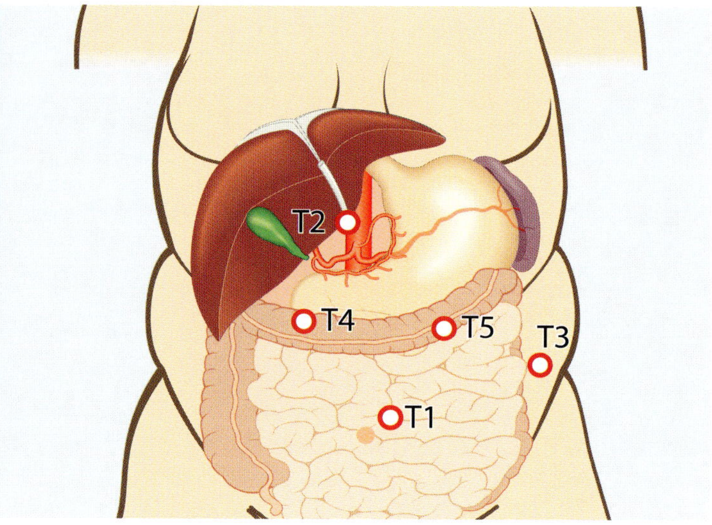

Insert an atraumatic forceps through T4. Occlude the proximal jejunum distal to the gastro-entero anastomosis.

Ask the anesthetist to fill the gastric tube with methylene blue solution until the pouch is stretched.

Watch for extravasation of dye while methylene blue is allowed to run into the pouch.

If no dye is monitored, the test is considered negative.

Note that a leak test is a security check. Always perform a leak test at the end of the operation, as the existence of a leak is hardly assessable without proper testing (→ p. 65, V-6).

Alternative: Performing an air test instead of the methylene blue test is also feasible. Occlude the intestine and ask the anesthetist to fill the gastric tube with air. Insert an irrigation device (T3) and supply saline solution. Watch for upcoming bubbles while oxygen is allowed to run into the pouch. If no bubbles are monitored, the test is considered negative.

Occluding the intestine

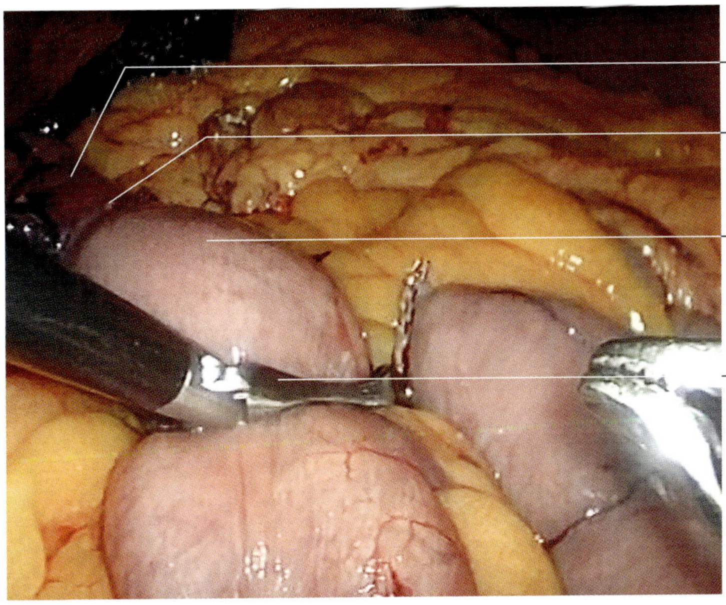

Gastric pouch

Gastro-entero anastomosis

Occluded intestine

Atraumatic forceps

Methylene blue filling of the gastro-entero anastomosis

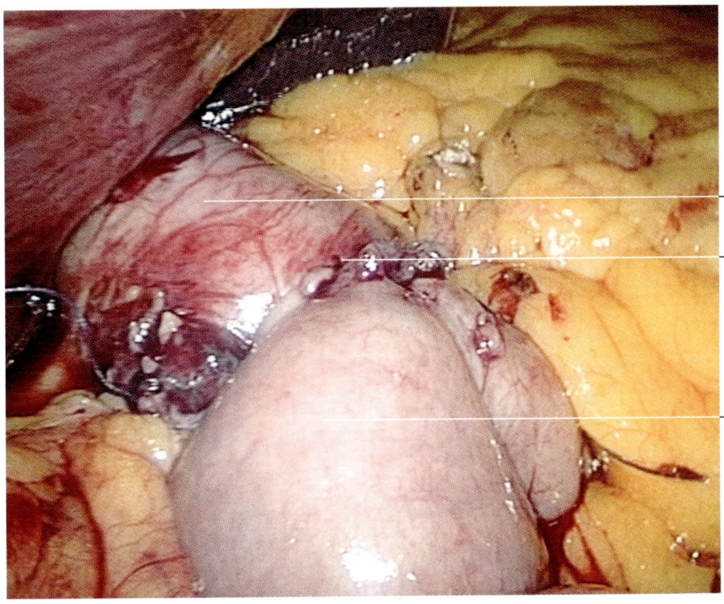

Gastric pouch (filled with methylene blue)

Gastro-entero anastomosis without extravasation

Intestine (filled with methylene blue)

Gastro-entero anastomosis filled with methylene blue solution

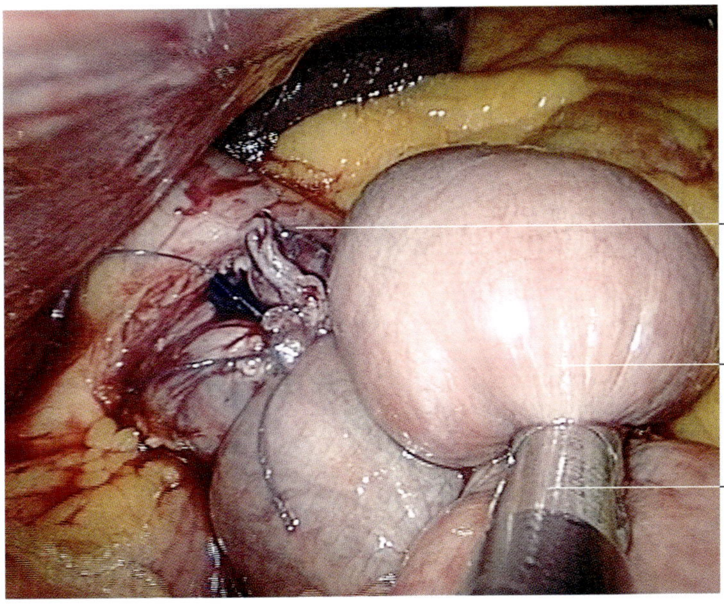

Gastric pouch (filled with methylene blue)

Intestine (filled with methylene blue)

Atraumatic forceps

13 Finishing the operation

T1 Scope
T2 –
T3 –
T4 Atraumatic forceps
T5 Atraumatic forceps, later Harmonic® ACE shears, if necessary

- Surgical forceps, needle holder, suture scissors and 2 Langenbeck hooks
- Fascia sutures 2–0 absorbable, polyfilament
- S.c. sutures 3–0 absorbable, polyfilament, if necessary
- Skin sutures 4–0 or 5–0 absorbable, monofilament or a skin stapler
- Dressings

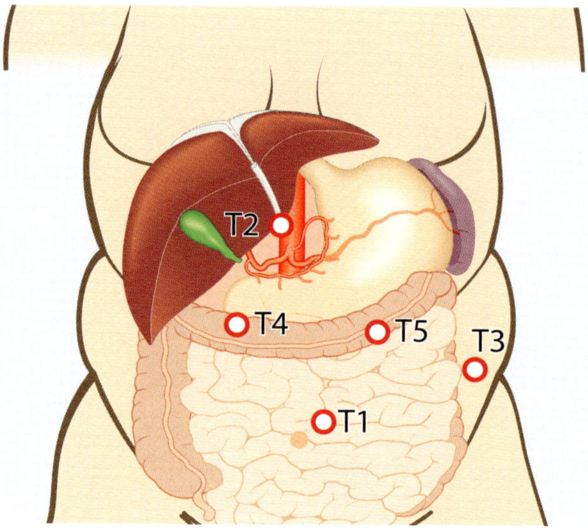

Inspect the operating field carefully and check for any bleeding and possible organ injuries. Stop any visible bleeding with the Harmonic® shears and treat any organ injury before continuing the operation.

In a routine setup with low risk patients and uncomplicated operations a drainage is usually not necessary. To reduce the risk in high risk patients, drainages may be advisable.

Remove the liver retracting device and the working trocars (T2–T5) carefully under vision.

Control the trocar incisions with regard to potential bleeding (→ p. 63, V-1; V-2).

Remove the scope (T1) and open the valve on the trocar for the scope for deflation. Then remove the trocar for the scope.

Close the fascia where 10/12 mm trocars have been introduced.

Close all incisions and cover the wounds with sterile dressings following disinfection.

Alternative: Instead of skin sutures and dressings Dermabond® (Ethicon Products) can be used to close the skin incisions.

Alternative: In high risk patients insert a silicone drain through T5. Grasp it with an atraumatic forceps (T4) and place it beyond the pouch. Insert a silicone drain through T3. Grasp it with an atraumatic forceps (T4) and place it beyond the entero-entero anastomosis.

Closed incisions

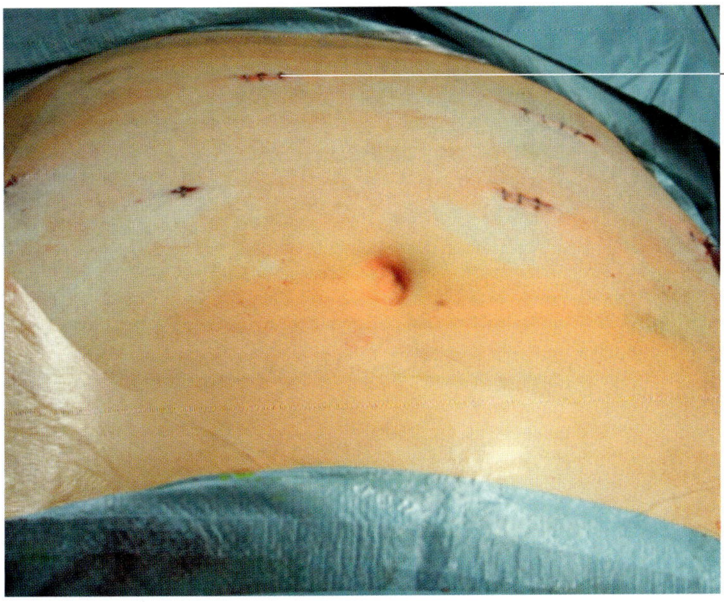

Closed port incision

Dressings

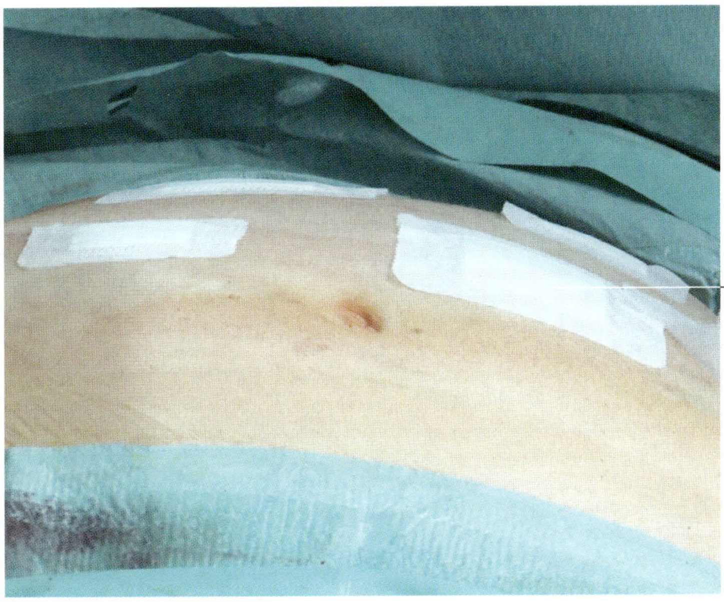

Adhesive sterile dressings

MANAGEMENT OF DIFFICULT SITUATIONS AND COMPLICATIONS

In principle, the decision to proceed to laparotomy should be made too early rather than too late! In obese patients, however, the possibility of other trocar positions should be considered before converting to a conventional operation in order to gain a better view! Convert immediately if the situation cannot be controlled laparoscopically!

1 Adhesions

Separate adhesions using the HF electrode, the ultrasonic device or curved scissors as close to the abdominal wall as possible so as not to injure any organs.

2 Blood vessel injuries

a) Diffuse bleeding/bleeding from minor vessels

Coagulate the bleeding vessel with the HF electrode or the ultrasonic device. If this does not terminate the bleeding, place a clip on the bleeding vessel.

Stop any bleeding close to the gastric wall, ideally with the HF electrode or the ultrasonic device or with an atraumatic transfixing suture.

b) Bleeding from major vessels

If large vessels such as the aorta, portal vein or vena cava are injured during the operation, open the abdomen immediately for vascular surgical treatment of the injury!

3 Organ injuries

In case of injuries where the extent cannot be determined with certainty, open the abdominal cavity for open management of the injury!

a) Greater omentum

Injury to the greater omentum can occur when the Veress needle is inserted too deeply and/or without elevation of the abdominal wall. All the safety tests may be positive, so that the complication can be identified only when the trocar for the scope and the scope are inserted.

Manage any bleeding that occurs with the HF electrode or the ultrasonic device. If, as a result of the insertion, the greater omentum is inflated like a tent, withdraw the trocar for the scope as far as the peritoneal margin and tap the abdomen with the flat hand. The omentum should then separate from the inside of the abdominal wall and collapse.

b) Esophagus

Injury to the esophagus is a very serious complication. Oversew the injury very carefully and then finish the operation without performing a gastric bypass procedure.

In case of an injury to the esophagus oversew the injury very carefully and do not perform a gastric bypass procedure!

c) Stomach

Perform gastroscopy to confirm a gastric injury and examine precisely where the lesion is located.

Oversew the lesion carefully with 1-0 absorbable material. Suturing of the defect can be done laparoscopically or in a conventional operation, depending on the extent of the lesion.

In case of staple line bleeding do not coagulate as it carries the risk of subsequent necrosis. Use clips or a suture to achieve a safe hemostasis.

d) Liver

Manage minor bleeding from the liver by brief compression with a swab or point contact with the Harmonic® shears.

In the case of major hemorrhage which can still be controlled laparoscopically, apply a hemostyptic.

e) Spleen

Bleeding from the spleen is ideally treated with the Harmonic® shears. Alternatively, apply a hemostyptic or perform a laparotomy, depending on the extension of the injury. Laparotomy is the exception.

f) Bowel

Bowel injuries are usually caused by instruments, especially by the Veress needle. Undissected adhesions can also be a cause of bowel injuries.

Manage bowel injuries by laparoscopic oversewing. If sufficient closure of the injury is not guaranteed, perform laparotomy. Irrigate the operating field gently with an antiseptic solution in order to reduce the risk of infection. As bowel resections always require a systemic antibiotic (single dose), the patient should already have antibiotic coverage (→ p. 19, I).

Staple line bleedings are not unusual. Don't coagulate any bleedings as it bears the risk of a necrosis subsequently. Use clips or a suture to achieve a safe hemostasis.

g) Pancreas

Manage minor bleeding from the pancreas by brief compression with a swab or point contact with Harmonic® shears.

In the case of major hemorrhage which can still be controlled laparoscopically, apply a hemostyptic.

To avoid pancreatic fistula it is recommended to insert a Penrose drain.

4 Preperitoneal air emphysema

a) Veress needle

If emphysema has occurred because of an incorrectly placed needle, remove the needle and reinsert it as previously described (→ p. 28, IIc). Ensure particularly that the angle of insertion is vertical and that the abdominal wall is lifted.

b) Trocar

Withdrawing a trocar so far that its opening comes to lie in front of the peritoneum is another cause of emphysema.

In this case, under direct vision, push the trocar back into the correct position through the existing incision.

5 Losing a swab in the abdominal cavity

After losing a swab, fix the trocar in its last position and, under direct vision, look for the swab where it was lost, using an atraumatic grasping forceps.

Do not change the patient's position, and do not irrigate the abdominal cavity!

If necessary, search for the swab with the C-arm or perform a laparotomy to retrieve the swab.

Do not give up searching until the swab is found!

6 Positive methylene blue leak test

If the leak test is positive, the anastomosis must be repaired or revised.

If the site of leakage is visible and is located on the anterior aspect of the anastomosis, place laparoscopic sutures for repair and repeat the leak test.

Anatomical variations

Sample operation note

Variation of the laparoscopic gastric bypass procedure: Circular stapler technique

3. Dividing the omentum
4. Creating the entero-entero anastomosis
5. Creating the access to the bursa
6. Stapling the stomach horizontally
7. Introducing the anvil of the circular stapler
8. Creating the gastro-entero anastomosis
9. Finalizing the gastric bypass

Postoperative management

a) Analgesia
b) Mobilization
c) Nutrition
d) Diagnostics
e) Medication
f) Discharge

Management of postoperative complications

a) Anastomotic leak
b) Anastomotic stricture
c) Gastro-gastric fistula
d) Internal herniation
e) Mixed upstream/downstream orientation of the anastomosis

Bibliography

Keywords

Editors

Assistants

Titles available

Anatomical variations

Accessory hepatic artery

In about 20 % of cases an accessory hepatic artery may be present in the region of the pars flaccida. Be aware of this possible anatomical variation when making the incision in the pars flaccida.

Sample operation note

Date:	Operating surgeon:
Patient's name:	Assistant:
Operation diagnosis: Morbid adipositas	Scrub nurse:
Operation: Laparoscopic Gastric Bypass	Anesthetist:

Patient under general anesthesia, placed in lithotomy position with adequate padding. Skin disinfection and sterile draping, followed by a skin incision about 15 cm below the xiphoid and 1–2 fingers paramedian on the left.

The Veress needle is inserted transmuscular through the incision and the usual safety tests are carried out. Pneumoperitoneum is then established with a pressure of 12 mmHg.

A 12 mm trocar for the scope is placed through this incision and the scope is brought into the abdomen. The patient is then placed in a reverse Trendelenburg position. A 360° view reveals no pathological changes and/or injuries. Under direct vision 5 mm trocar is placed in the right upper abdomen and the liver retracting device is inserted and fixed with the self-retainer.

Then one 5 mm and two 12 mm trocars are placed in the left lateral abdomen and in the right and left epigastrium, respectively, under vision.

The angle of His is dissected using Harmonic® shears. The lesser omentum is incised at the lesser curvature of the stomach, caudal to the gastro-esophageal junction. Then the omental bursa is explored and dissected in the direction of the left crus of the diaphragm.

The gastric calibration tube is inserted and placed in the cardia by the anesthetist. The tube is filled with 25 ml saline solution.

A gastric pouch is created by using an endoscopic linear cutter and a gastrotomy is performed by incising the horizontal staple line.

The ligament of Treitz is indentified and a jejunal distance of 20–50 cm is measured. Then an enterotomy is performed and the intestine is connected to the pouch using the endoscopic linear cutter. The remaining opening of the gastro-entero anastomosis is closed by placing one interrupted and one single layer running suture.

Starting from the pouch an intestinal distance of 120 cm is measured and an enterotomy is performed. An additional enterotomy is performed at the distal part of the (future) bilio-pancreatic limb at a distance of 3–5 cm to the gastric pouch. The intestine is connected to the (future) bilio-pancreatic limb using the endoscopic linear cutter. The remaining opening of the entero-entero anastomosis is closed by placing one interrupted and one single layer running suture.

The intestine is divided between the gastric pouch and the entero-entero anastomosis using an endoscopic linear cutter. The linear cutter is placed close to the pouch.

The gastro-entero anastomosis is tested for leaks; then the gastric calibration tube is removed by the anesthetist.

Following inspection of the operating field, the trocars are removed. The incisions are closed and covered with sterile dressings.

APPENDICES

Variation of the laparoscopic gastric bypass procedure: Circular stapler technique

01 Exploring the abdominal cavity

02 Identifying the anatomical landmarks

03 Dividing the omentum

04 Creating the entero-entero anastomosis

05 Creating the access to the bursa

06 Stapling the stomach horizontally

07 Introducing the anvil of the circular stapler

08 Creating the gastro-entero anastomosis

09 Finalizing the gastric bypass

12 Testing the gastro-entero anastomosis for leaks

13 Finishing the operation

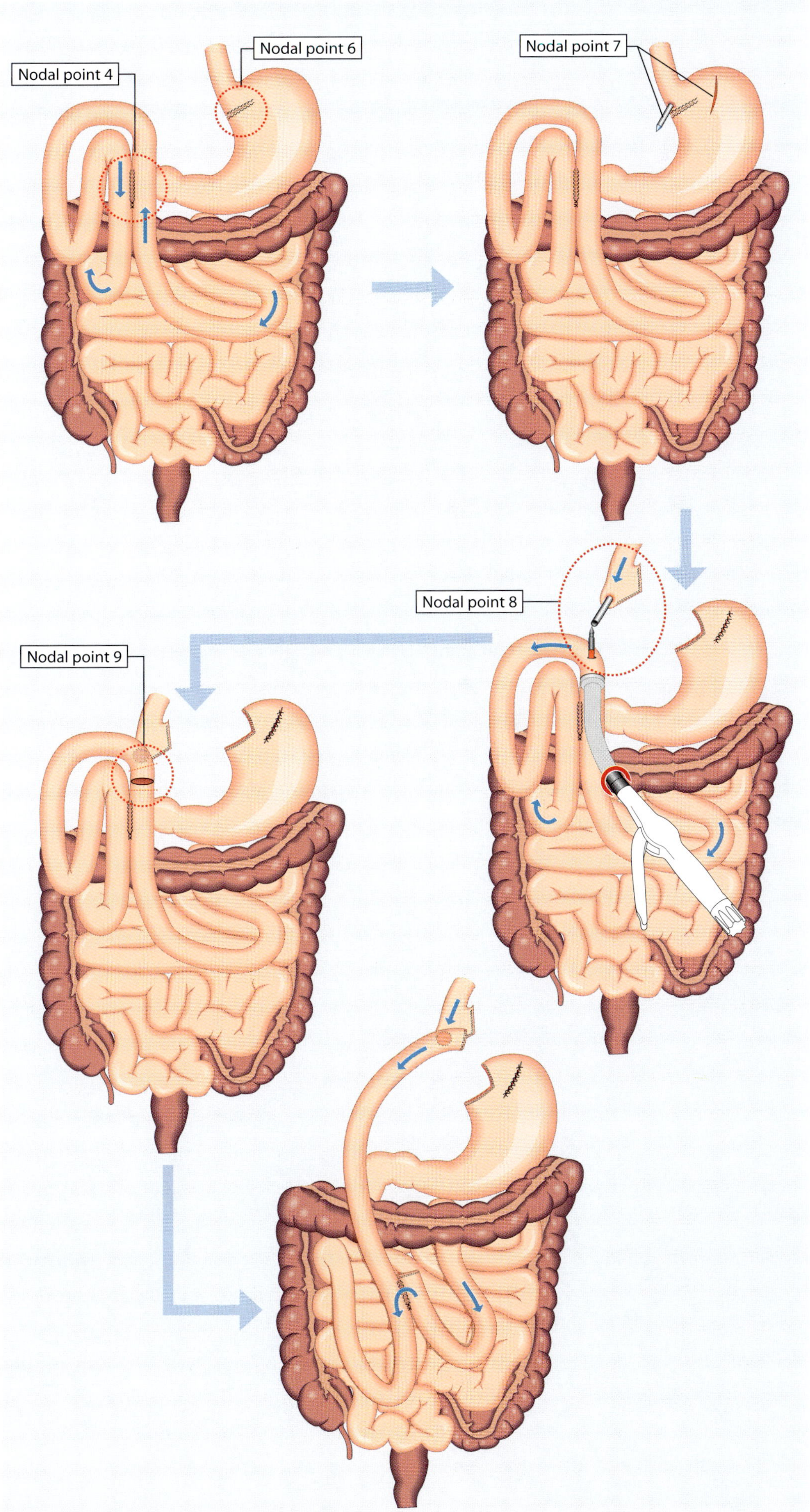
Nodal point 6
Nodal point 4
Nodal point 7
Nodal point 8
Nodal point 9

Variation of the laparoscopic gastric bypass procedure: Circular stapler technique

Perform nodal points 1 and 2 as described on page 34–37.

Exploring the abdominal cavity
Identifying the anatomical landmarks
Dividing the omentum
Creating the entero-entero anastomosis
Creating the access to the bursa
Stapling the stomach horizontally
Introducing the anvil of the circular stapler
Creating the gastro-entero anastomosis
Finalizing the gastric bypass
Testing the gastro-entero anastomosis for leaks
Finishing the operation

3 Dividing the omentum

T1 Scope
T2 Liver retracting device
T3 Atraumatic grasping forceps (assistant)
T4 Atraumatic grasping forceps
T5 Harmonic® shears

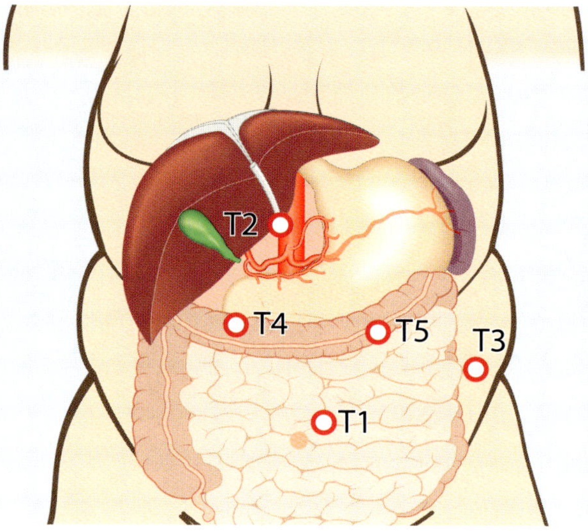

Dividing the greater omentum simplifies the mobilization of the proximal jejunum.

Have the assistant grasp the greater omentum with an atraumatic forceps (T3) and pull it laterally to the left.

Grasp the greater omentum with a second atraumatic forceps (T4), pull it laterally to the right.

Divide the omentum in cranial direction using the Harmonic® shears (T5), aiming from the level of T5 towards the pouch. Divide the omentum up to the transverse colon and leave the gastrocolic ligament intact. Take care not to injure the blood-supplying vessels of the colon (→ p. 63, V-2, V-3).

Take care not to injure the colon's blood-supplying vessels or the gastro-epiploic artery while dividing the omentum.

Dividing the omentum

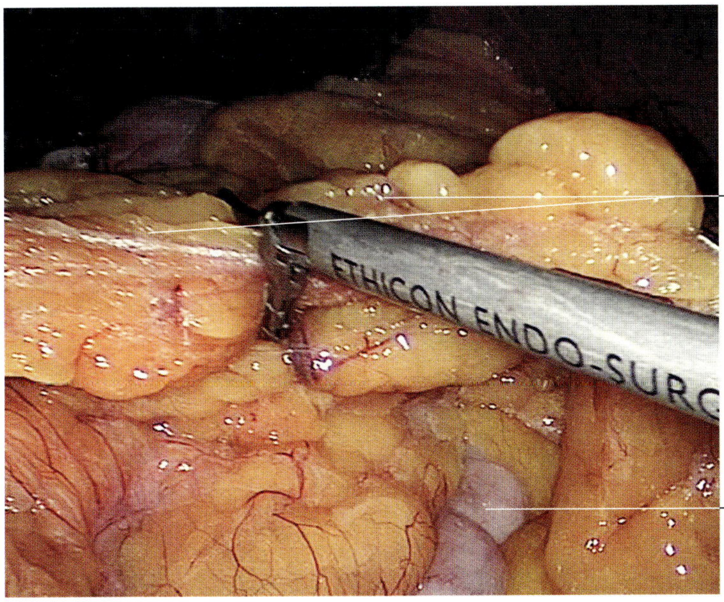

Dividing the omentum up to the transverse colon

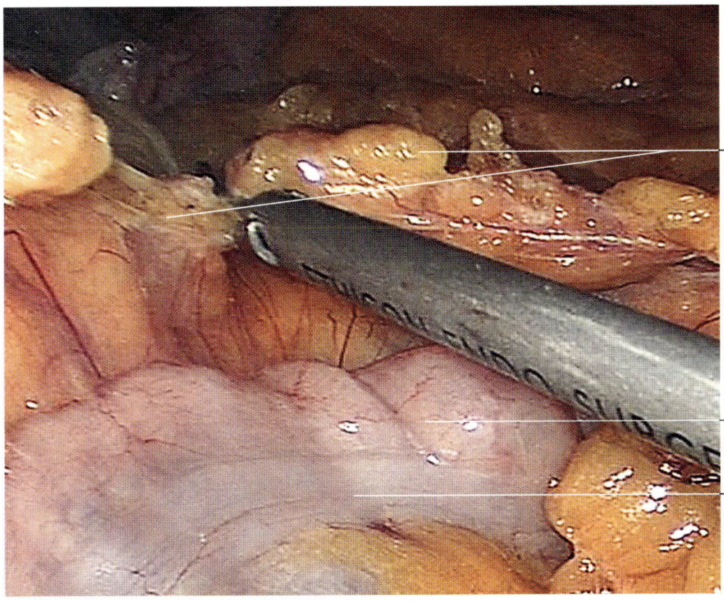

4 Creating the entero-entero anastomosis

T1 Scope
T2 Liver retracting device
T3 Atraumatic grasping forceps (assistant)
T4 Atraumatic grasping forceps
T5 Atraumatic forceps with landmark, later Harmonic® shears, later endoscopic linear cutter, later needle holder

- Different cartridges (depending on tissue thickness)
- Absorbable sutures 3–0 (e.g. Vicryl™)

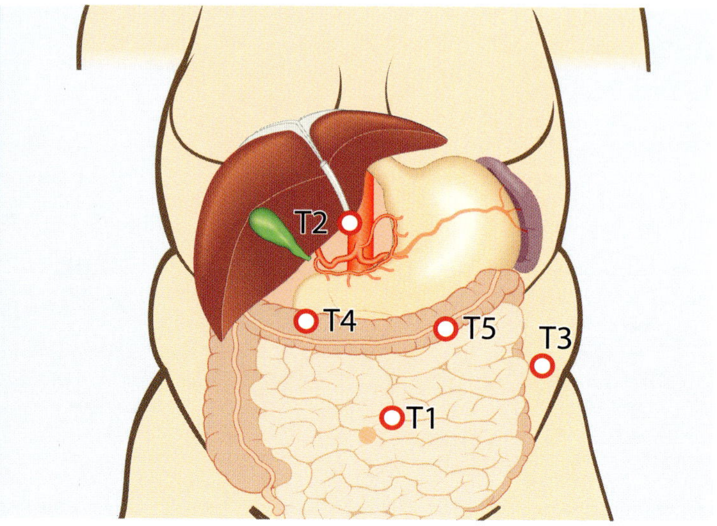

Grasp the intestine with atraumatic forceps (T4 and T5) at the ligament of Treitz and measure step by step a distance of 50 cm in downstream direction and place a marker clip. Subsequently, measure a distance of 120–150 cm from the marked intestinal part in downstream direction. There is a lack of consensus and no hard evidence for deciding on the length of the alimentary limb. The authors usually prefer a length of 120 cm.

Remove the atraumatic forceps from T5 and insert it through T3. Have the assistant grasp the intestine with the atraumatic forceps (T3). Perform an enterotomy in the measured distal intestine using the Harmonic® shears (T5).

Grasp the future bilio-pancreatic limb near to the marker clip with an atraumatic forceps (T4) and perform a second enterotomy using the Harmonic® shears (T5).

Place the enterotomy of the future alimentary limb beside the enterotomy of the future bilio-pancreatic limb. Take care that the two limbs have antiparallel upstream/downstream orientation.

Take care that the two limbs have antiparallel upstream/downstream orientation **(→ p. 87, appendices).**

Insert the endoscopic linear cutter (T5) loaded with white or blue cartridges (1.0/1.5 mm closed staple height), depending on the thickness of the intestinal wall.

To create a side to side anastomosis, place the stapler anvil into the opening of the future alimentary limb in an upstream direction and place the stapler cartridge into the future bilio-pancreatic limb in a downstream direction.

Close the endoscopic linear cutter.

Prior to firing, keep the linear cutter closed for about 15 seconds. Accurate tissue compression minimizes the tissue liquid and ensures proper and safe stapling.

Fire the endoscopic linear cutter. Open the jaws of the endoscopic linear cutter.

Perform a second firing with the endoscopic linear cutter in downstream direction to ensure a sufficient diameter of the entero-entero anastomosis.

Insert a needle holder with a 3–0 absorbable thread (T5) and close the enterostoma with a running suture.

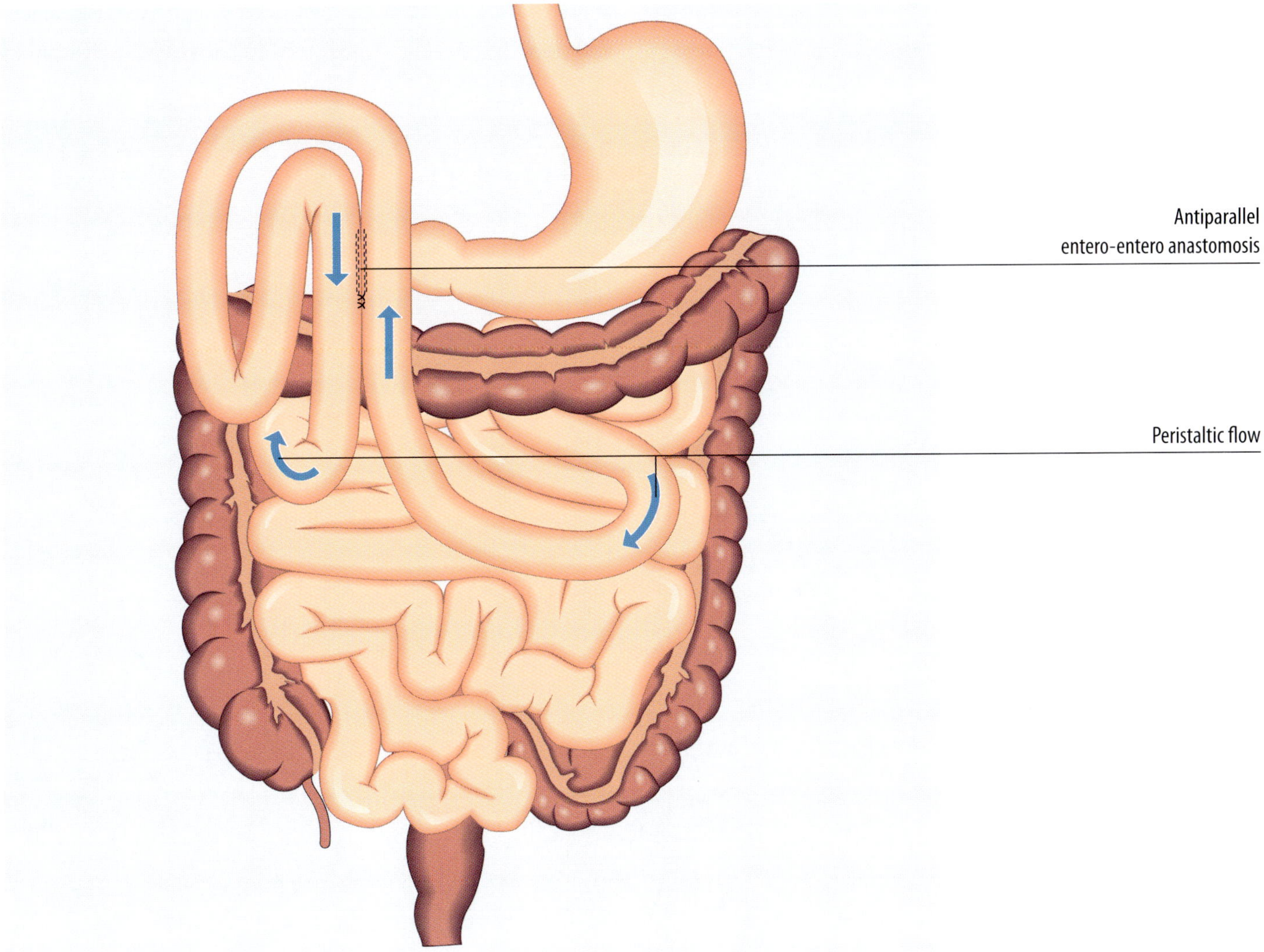
Antiparallel
entero-entero anastomosis
Peristaltic flow

5 Creating the access to the bursa

T1	Scope
T2	Liver retracting device
T3	Atraumatic grasping forceps (assistant)
T4	Harmonic® shears
T5	Atraumatic grasping forceps

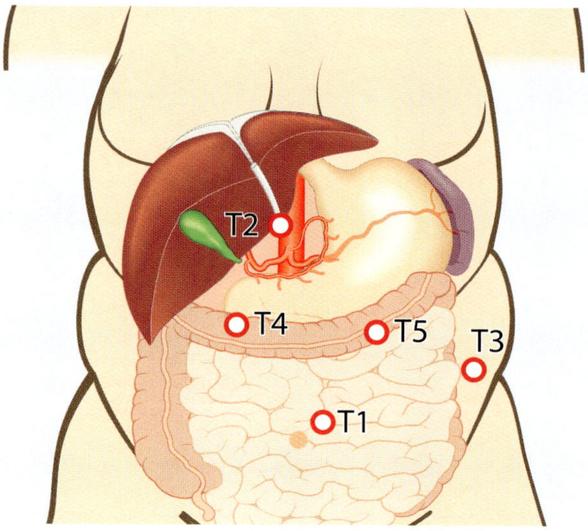

Grasp the fundus with an atraumatic forceps (T5) and pull it down to visualize the left crus of the diaphragm. Free the angle of His using the Harmonic® shears (T4) to reduce tension on the stomach.

Dissect the angle of His to reduce the tension on the stomach and to avoid injuries.

Have the assistant grasp the fundus and pull it laterally to the left (T3). Use the Harmonic® shears (T4) and open the omental bursa close to the lesser curvature approximately 4 cm distal to the cardia. Push the lesser curvature laterally and ventrally by using the atraumatic forceps (T5). Dissect the lesser curvature towards the gastro-esophageal junction. Take care not to injure the left gastric artery, as it assures the blood supply to the pouch (→ p. 63, V-2a).

Dissect close to the gastric wall and take care not to injure the left gastric artery as it assures the blood supply to the pouch.

Perform a retrogastric dissection by exploring the bursa. Use the Harmonic® shears (T4) and dissect layer for layer, carefully and under vision. Dissect in the direction of the left crus of the diaphragm.

Work under vision control to avoid any injuries to the gastric wall, spleen or other tissue.

Creating the access to the bursa

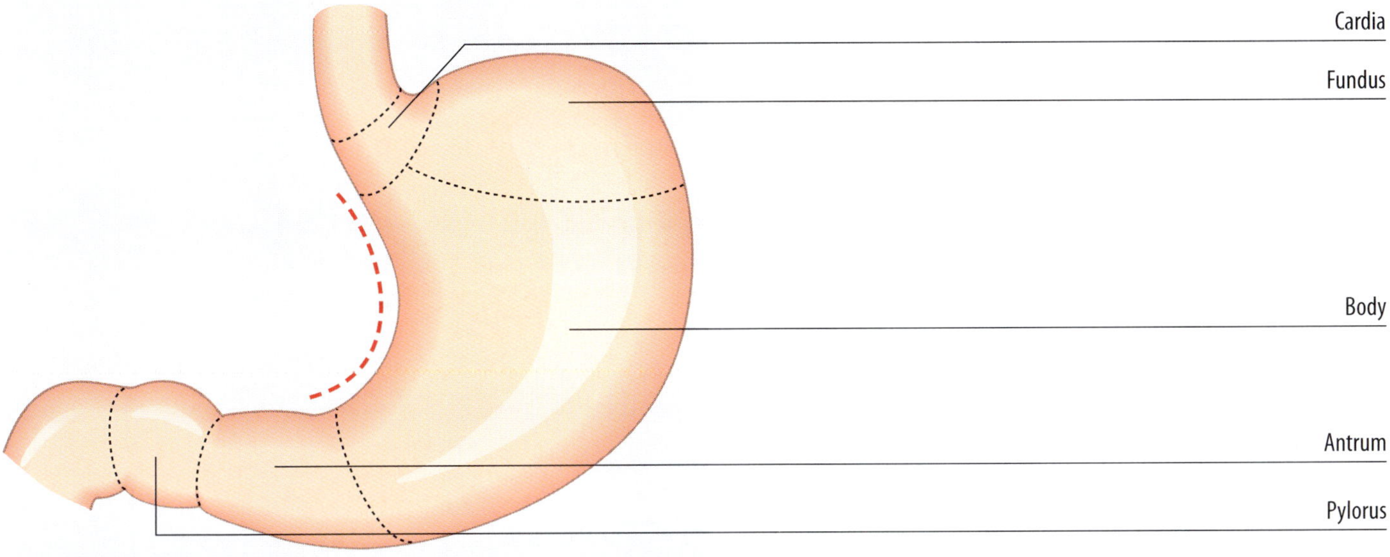

Opening the bursa

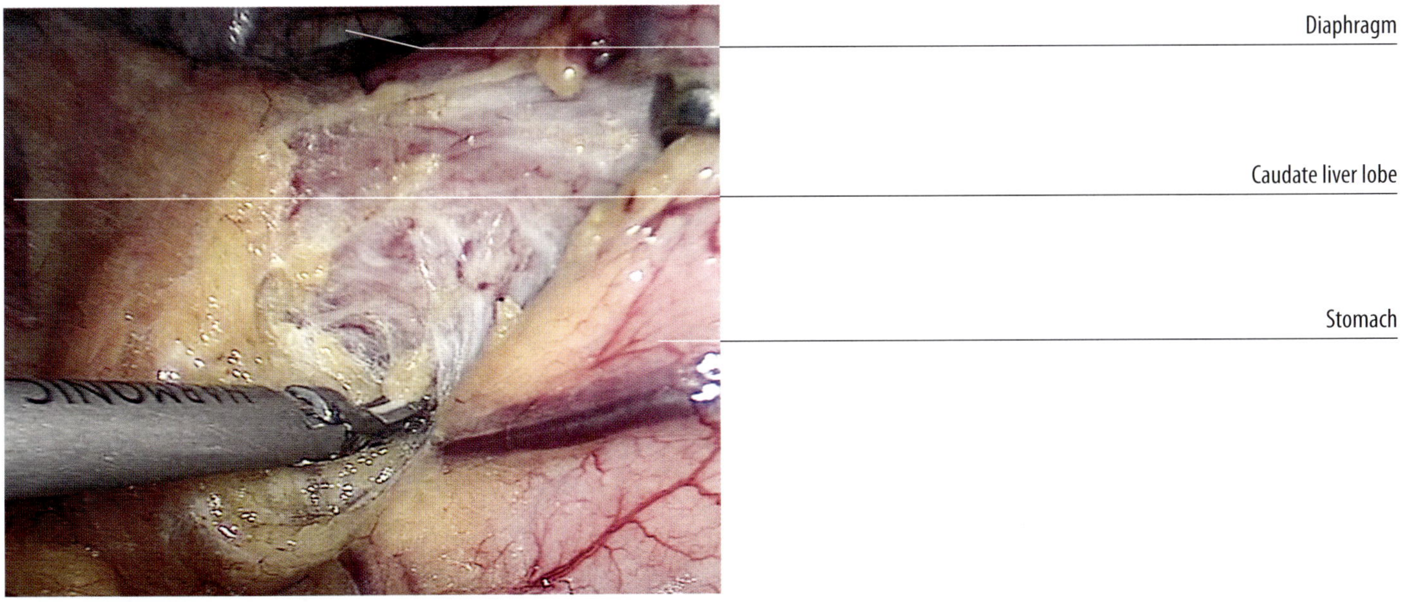

Access to the bursa

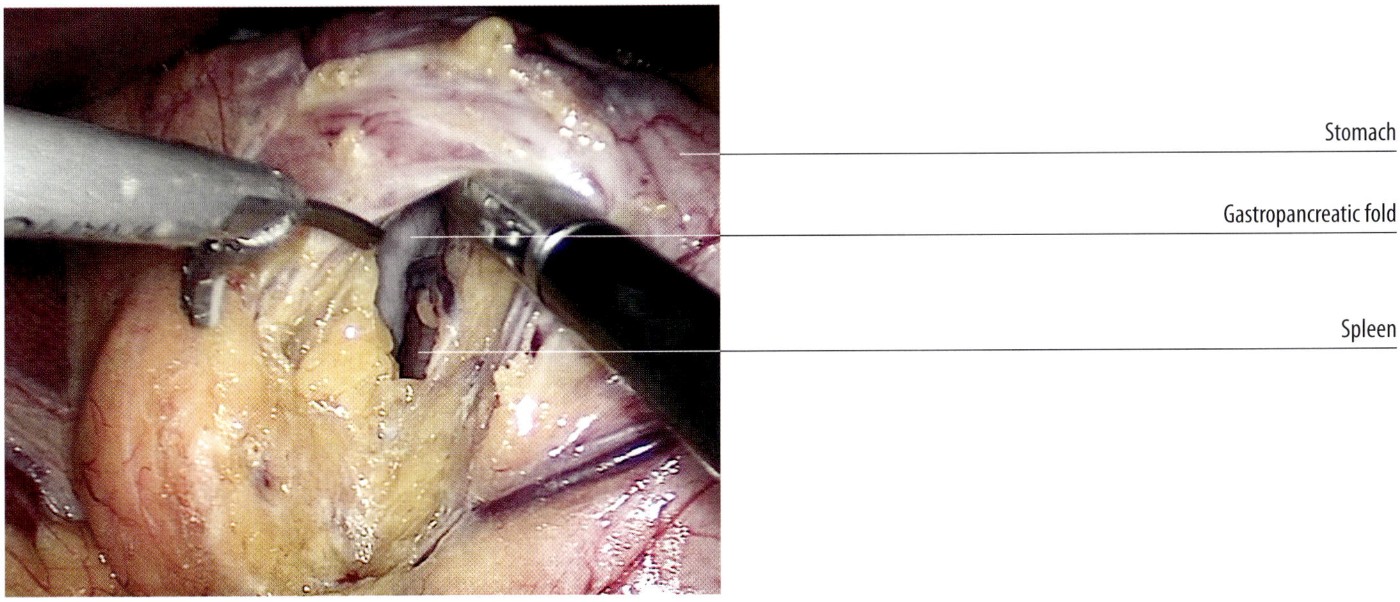

6 Stapling the stomach horizontally

T1 Scope
T2 Liver retracting device
T3 Atraumatic grasping forceps (assistant)
T4 Endoscopic linear cutter (45 mm cutter length)
T5 Atraumatic grasping forceps

– Different cartridges (depending on tissue thickness)

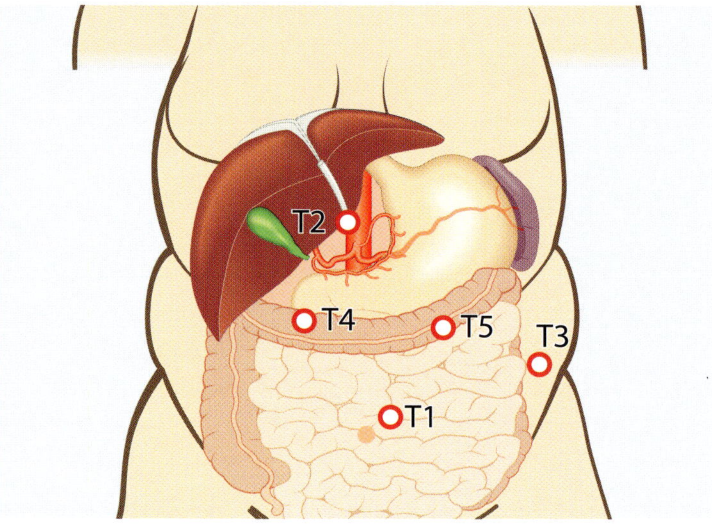

Use a gastric calibration tube with a balloon to ensure an optimal calibration of the pouch size.

Ask the anesthetist to pass the gastric calibration tube into the stomach and to slowly fill the balloon of the tube with 25 ml saline solution. Then tell him to draw the tube back into the cardia.

Note that the pouch size is less than 30 ml to ensure an adequate weight loss postoperatively.

Have the assistant insert an atraumatic forceps into the opened bursa behind the stomach (T3) to lift it ventrally.

Grasp the lesser curvature at the corpus with an atraumatic forceps (T5).

Insert the endoscopic linear cutter (T4) and place it horizontally below the cardia. Use gold or green cartridges (1.8/2.0 mm closed staple height) for the division of the stomach, depending on the thickness of the stomach wall.

Before closing the linear cutter be sure not to overtighten the stomach. This may cause an insufficient distance to the cardia.

Close the endoscopic linear cutter. In case of difficulty with closing the cutter, adjust the positioning of the jaws and grasp less tissue. An accumulation of tissue at the proximal end of the jaws may result in an incomplete staple line.

Take care not to accumulate tissue at the proximal jaws as this may result in an incomplete staple line.

Prior to firing, keep the endoscopic linear cutter closed for about 15 seconds. The accurate tissue compression minimizes the tissue liquid and ensures a proper staple formation and a safe staple line.

Fire the endoscopic linear cutter. Usually it is sufficient to create the horizontal staple line with 1 firing.

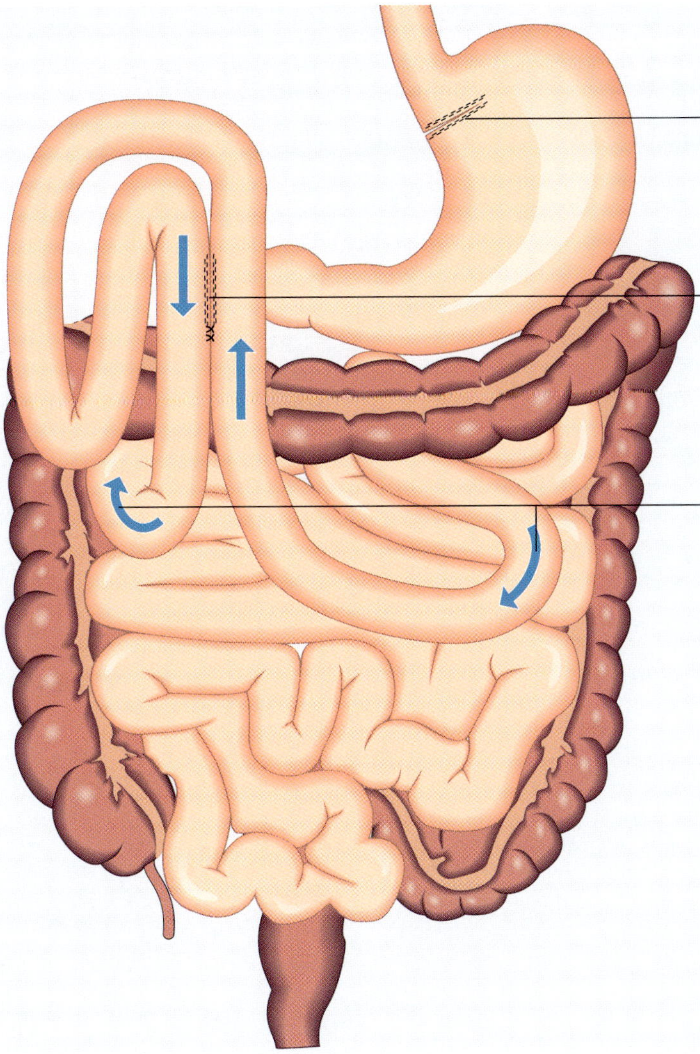
Horizontal staple line
Antiparallel entero-entero anastomosis
Peristaltic flow

Variation of the laparoscopic gastric bypass procedure: Circular stapler technique

7 Introducing the anvil of the circular stapler

T1 Scope
T2 Liver retracting device
T3 –
T4 Atraumatic grasping forceps
T5 Harmonic® shears, later anvil forceps, later endoscopic linear cutter, later needle holder

– Absorbable sutures 3–0 (e.g. Vicryl™)

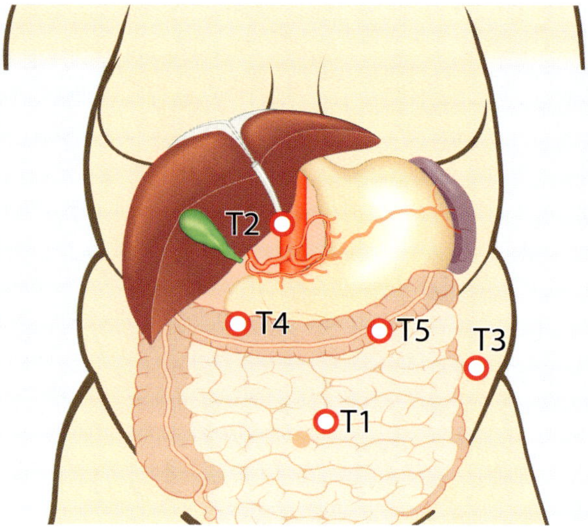

Perform a gastrotomy with Harmonic® shears (T5) by incising the fundus lateral to the staple line.

Take care not to affect the horizontal staple line while performing the gastrotomy with Harmonic® shears.

Insert the anvil with the attached anvil shaft into the stomach through the gastrotomy.

Perforate the gastric pouch with the attached anvil shaft in its right lateral part above the staple line. Grasp the anvil shaft with the anvil forceps (T5).

Introduce the endoscopic linear cutter (T5). Divide the gastric pouch towards the angle of His until the stomach is completely divided.

Insert a needle holder with a 3–0 absorbable thread (T5) and close the gastrotomy with a running suture.

Placed anvil in the cardia

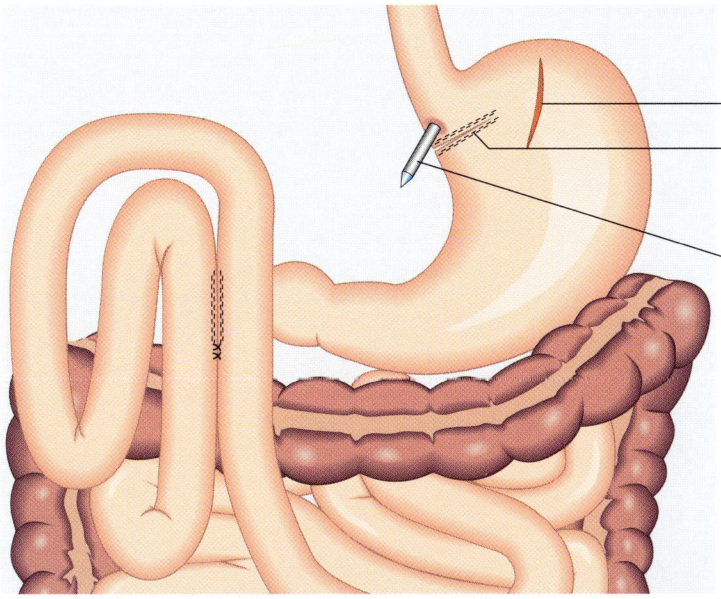

Gastrotomy

Horizontal staple line

Anvil with shaft

Inserting the circular stapler's anvil into the pouch

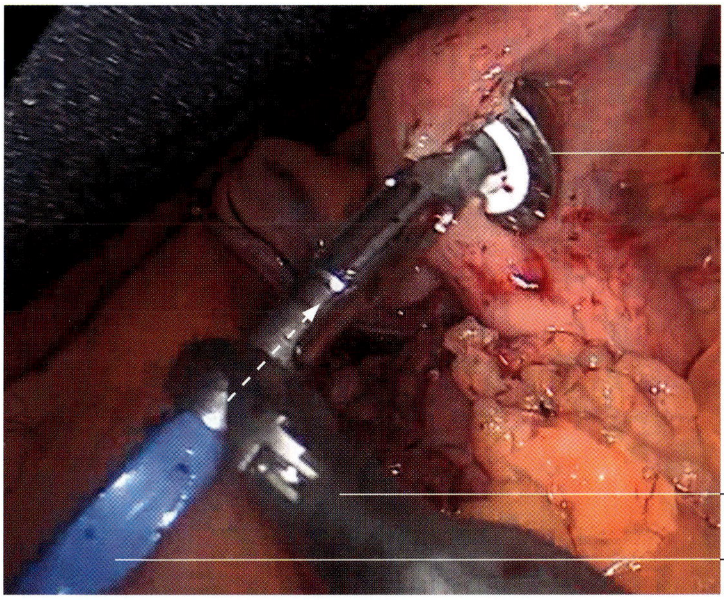

Anvil is placed through gastrotomy

Anvil forceps

Anvil shaft

Perforating the gastric pouch

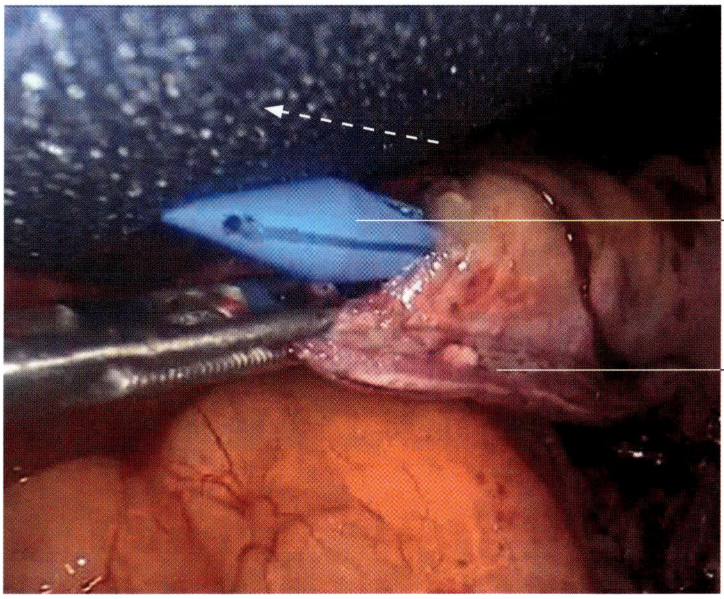

Anvil shaft

Horizontal staple line

Variation of the laparoscopic gastric bypass procedure: Circular stapler technique

8 Creating the gastro-entero anastomosis

T1 Scope
T2 Liver retracting device
T3 –
T4 Atraumatic grasping forceps, later anvil forceps
T5 Harmonic® shears, later endoscopic circular stapler

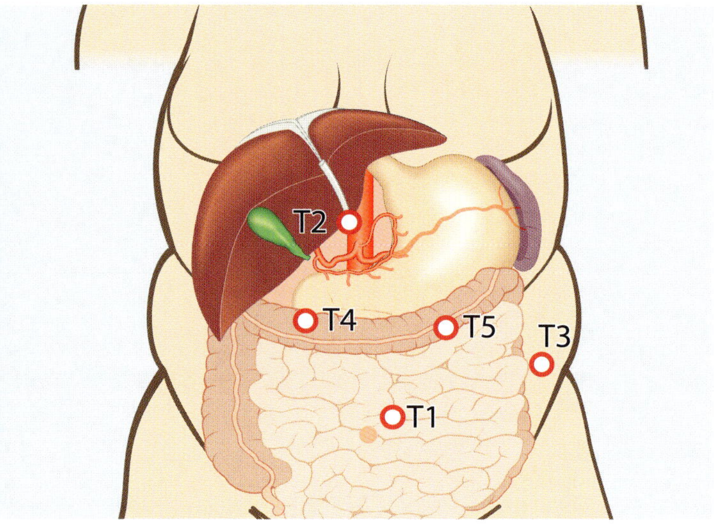

Insert the Harmonic® shears (T5) and incise the (future) alimentary limb at its proximal part at a distance of 4–5 cm to the entero-entero anastomosis.

Insert the circular stapler (T5) into the performed enterotomy in a downstream direction.

Perforate the intestine with the trocar shaft of the circular stapler. Connect the anvil shaft to the trocar shaft of the circular stapler using the anvil forceps (T4).

Anastomose the gastric pouch with the jejunum.

Remove the circular stapler.

Creating the gastro-entero anastomosis

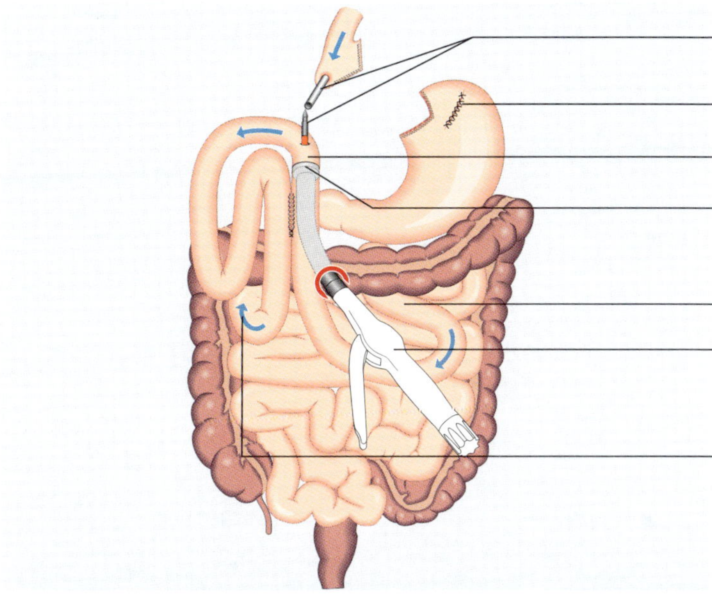

Inserting the circular stapler through the jejunostomy

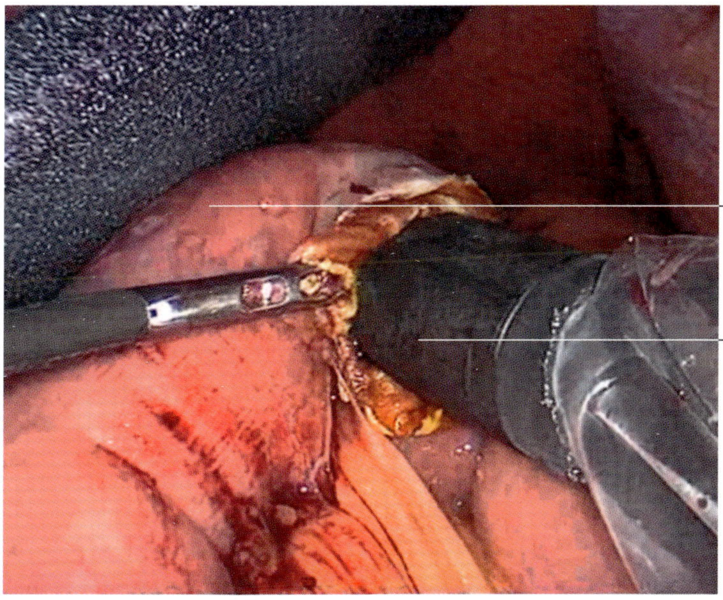

Anastomosing the gastric pouch with the jejunum

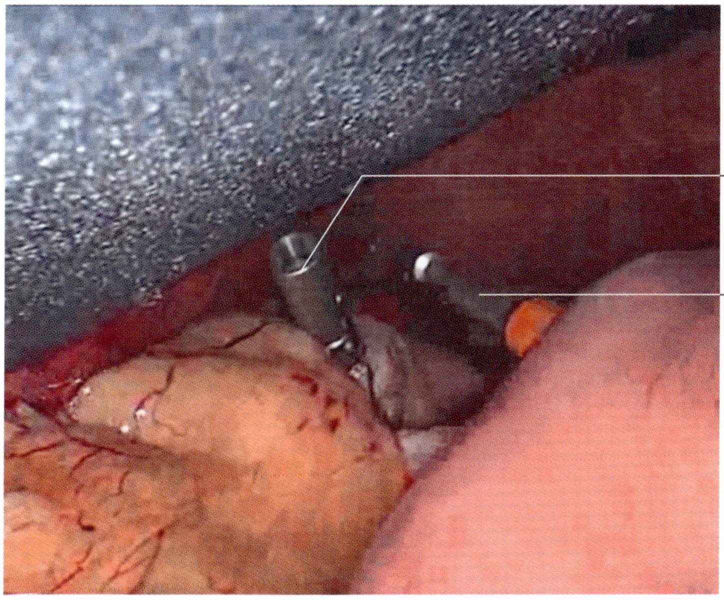

9 Finalizing the gastric bypass

T1 Scope
T2 Liver retracting device
T3 –
T4 Atraumatic grasping forceps, later endoscopic linear stapler
T5 Harmonic® shears, later atraumatic grasping forceps, later needle holder

– Retrieval pouch
– Non-absorbable sutures 2–0 (e.g. Ethibond™ excel)

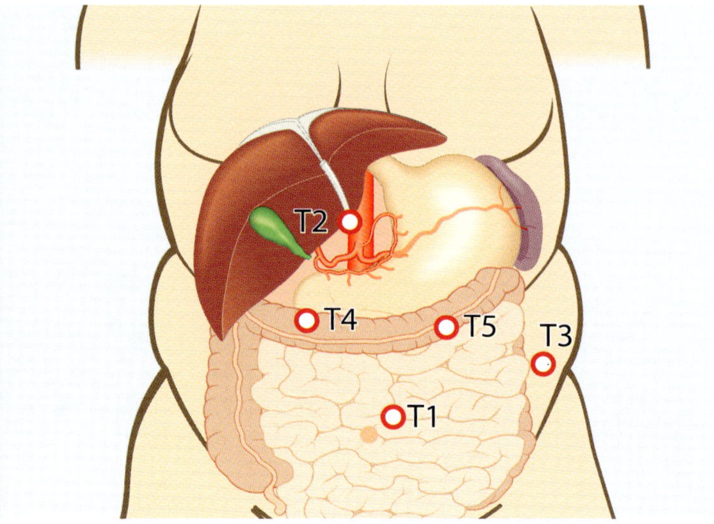

Incise the mesentery at the level of the enterotomy with Harmonic® shears (T5). Dissect the intestine proximal and distal to the enterotomy.

Transect the intestine proximal and distal to the enterotomy using the endoscopic linear cutter (T4).

Insert the resected intestine into a retrieval pouch and remove it from the abdominal cavity.

Insert a needle holder with a 2–0 non-absorbable thread (T5) and close the mesentery defect with a running suture.

Perform a leak test of the gastro-entero anastomosis with methylene blue solution as described on page 58–59 and finish the operation as described on page 60–61.

Stapling lines proximal and distal to the enterotomy

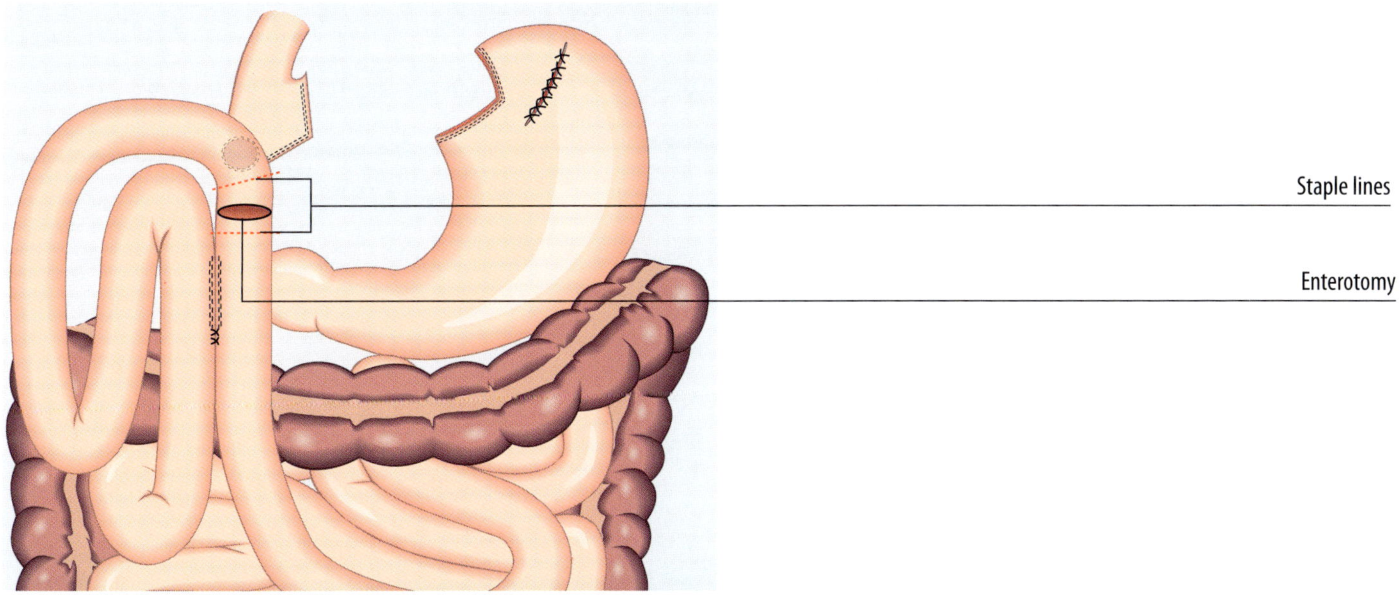

Stapling distal to the enterotomy

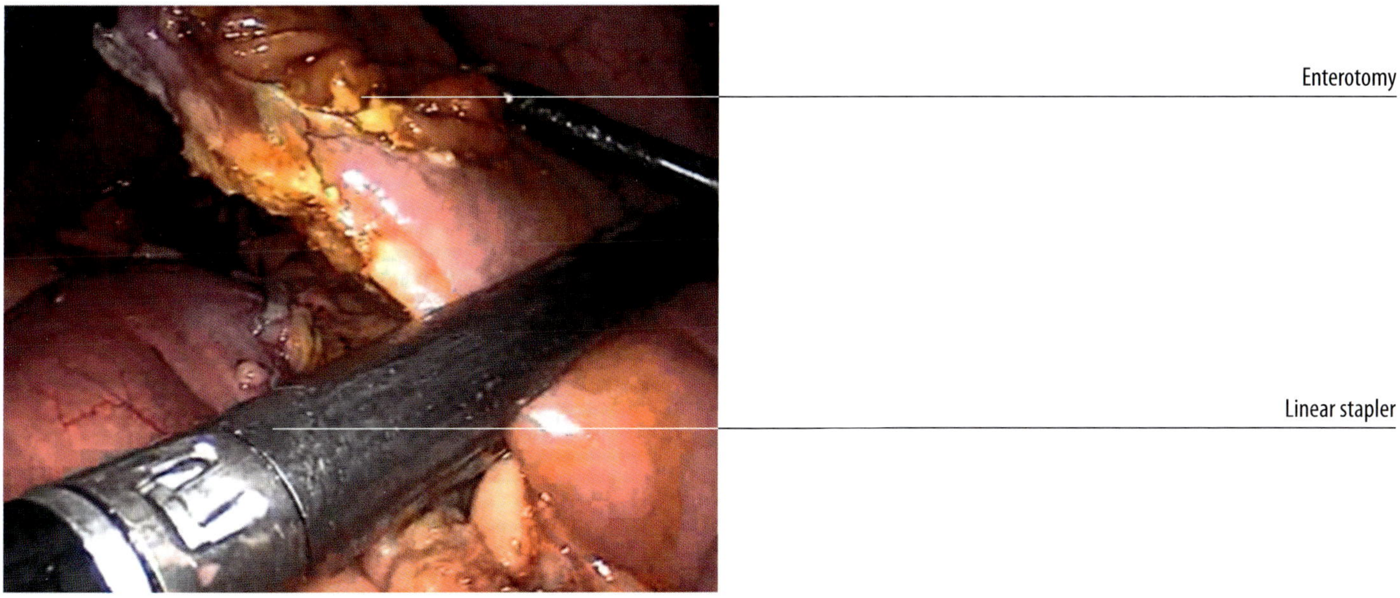

Created gastric bypass

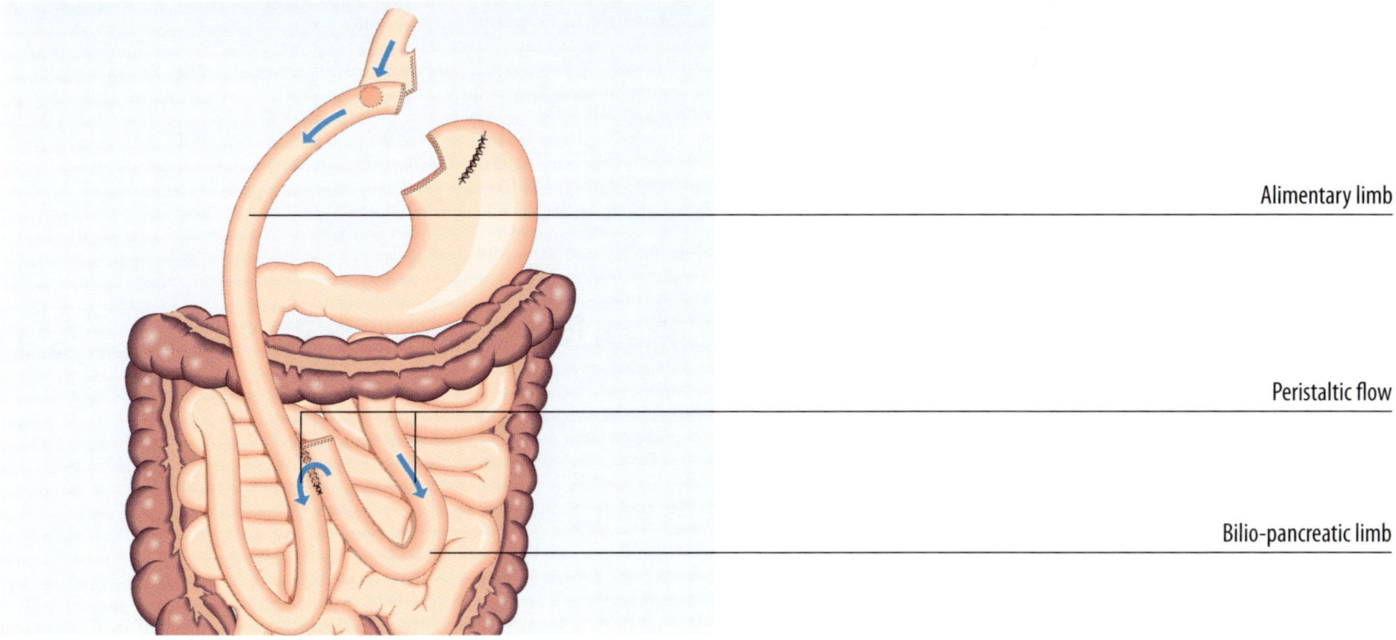

Postoperative management

a) Analgesia

Take care to give adequate pain medication for fast recovery of the patient.

On day of operation give opioids as needed by the patient. From the first postoperative day prescription of simple analgesia (NSAIDs) is sufficient in most cases.

b) Mobilization

Depending on anesthetic aftereffects and circulatory stability, mobilize the patient as soon as possible postoperatively. Try to do so on the evening of the operation.

c) Nutrition

Reintroduction of food differs from hospital to hospital. Our recommendation is the following:

First and second postoperative day: Nourish the patient parenterally and give him a limited volume of fluids orally.

Third postoperative day: Start with fluid food (soup, drinkable yoghurt, ...).

Continue the fluid diet for 3-4 weeks. Begin with first solid food after 4 weeks.

d) Diagnostics

Take blood samples and control the vital signs regularly. This enables to detect a tachycardia quite early. Tachycardia predominates as the first sign of sepsis in postoperative bariatric patients.

The classic signs or symptoms of sepsis such as abdominal pain, fever, or leukocytosis often occur at a later time.

In case of tachycardia over 120 bpm a re-laparoscopy should be considered.

Performing an X-ray with Gastrografin postoperatively on a routine basis is a matter of controversy. If a multi-step operation series is planned we recommend postoperative monitoring of the anastomosis via X-ray.

e) Medication

Medication should consist of gastric acid inhibitors (PPI) for about 2 weeks and low-molecular-weight heparin for anticoagulation combined with graded elastic compression stockings during hospitilization. If the patient is known to have diabetes mellitus, measure the blood glucose level continuously; you may need to reduce the required insulin units quite soon after operation. Supply vitamin B12 parenterally every 3 months.

f) Discharge

Patients considered to be at low risk may be discharged on the second postoperative day, provided that they are pain free, able to drink 1500 ml/24 hours, have no fever, and can handle all activities of daily life.

Management of postoperative complications

a) Anastomotic leak

A leak occurs most often at the gastro-entero anastomosis. It is essential to detect an insufficiency of the anastomosis very early to prevent sepsis and a potential life-threatening situation. Any heartbeat rate over 120 bpm should be considered to be caused by sepsis and should give rise to consideration of a revision.

This complication usually occurs within the first 24 postoperative hours. Typically, the first symptom is a rapid pulse.

Tachycardia exceeding 120 bpm in the early postoperative hours is a sign of sepsis and an indication for emergency laparoscopy.

Obese patients show the classic signs of a sepsis as a worsening abdominal pain, fever, or leukocytosis later than patients with a normal BMI. Symptoms of stomach leak also include dizziness and a shortness of breath.

Re-perform a laparoscopy within the first 36 hours after surgery if a leak is suspected; locate the leak with the methylene blue test and oversew it meticulously. Longer persisting leaks should be treated with a stent and a local drainage. Early detection of a leak is essential to prevent the development of sepsis.

b) Anastomotic stricture

Anastomotic stricture can happen immediately after surgery (secondarily caused by ischemia or edema) or in the course of time (most often caused by adhesions). It commonly occurs at the gastro-entero anastomosis.

Typical clinical signs include epigastric pain, early satiety, vomiting, and also tachycardia.

Acute gastric distension recognized via X-ray is always a sign of an obstruction. Stomach distension carries the risk of staple line leakage.

Gastroenteral strictures can often be diagnosed and treated by gastroscopy.

c) Gastro-gastric fistula

The characteristic sign of a gastro-gastric fistula is an early cessation of the initial weight loss followed by weight gain.

If a gastro-gastric fistula is detected, plan selective surgery. The only way to ensure persistent weight loss lies in a surgical intervention.

d) Internal herniation

Internal hernia occurs more often after retrocolic gastric bypass than after an antecolic bypass procedure. Also it seems that longer bilio-pancreatic limbs predispose to a higher rate of herniations.

Closure of internal hernias may be indicated, although the incidence of internal herniations is very low at some institutions. Moreover, closure of the internal spaces does not totally preclude the risk of future herniation.

e) Mixed upstream/downstream orientation of the anastomosis

In case of mixed-up loops the operative revision has to be done immediately (< 36 hours), otherwise a cardiac arrest would occur in the early postoperative phase due to an over-stretched stomach (distension).

Bibliography

Arasaki C.H., Del Grande J.C., Yanagita E.T., Alves A.K. & Oliveira D.R. (2005). Incidence of regurgitation after the banded gastric bypass. *Obesity Surgery,* 15: 1408–1417.

Arora S., Aggarwal R., Sevdalis N., Moran A., Sirimanna P., Kneebone R. & Darzi A. (2010). Development and validation of mental practice as a training strategy for laparoscopic surgery. *Surgical Endoscopy,* 24: 179–187.

Baker R.S., Foote J., Kemmeter P., Brady R., Vroegop T. & Serveld M. (2004). The science of stapling and leaks. Review. *Obesity Surgery*, 14: 1290–1298.

Boru C. & Silecchia G. (2010). Bariatric emergencies: what the general surgeon should know. *Chirurgia (Bucur),* 105: 455–464.

Brolin R.E., Kenler H.A., Gorman J.H. & Cody R.P. (1992). Long-limb gastric bypass in the super-obese. A prospective randomized study. *Annals of Surgery,* 215: 387–395.

Carpenter W.B. (1874). *Principles of Mental Physiology: With their Applications to the Training and Discipline of the Mind and the Study of its Comorbid Conditions.* London: Henry S. King & Co.

Choban P.S. & Flancbaum L. (2002). The effect of Roux limb lengths on outcome after Roux-en-Y gastric bypass: a prospective, randomized clinical trial. *Obesity Surgery,* 12: 540–545.

Elariny H., Gonzalez H. & Wang B. (2005). Tissue thickness of human stomach measured on excised gastric specimens of obese patients. *Surgical Technology International,* 14: 119–124.

Feltz D.L. & Landers D.M. (1983). The effects of mental practice on motor skill learning and performance: a meta-analysis. *Journal of Sport Psychology,* 5: 25–57.

Fobi M.A., Lee H., Felahy B., Che-Senge K., Fields C.B. & Sanguinette M.C. (2005). Fifty consecutive patients with the GaBP ring system used in the banded gastric bypass operation for obesity with follow up of at least 1 year. *Surgery for Obesity and Related Diseases,* 1: 569–572.

Griffen W.O. Jr., Young V.L. & Stevenson C.C. (1977). A prospective comparison of gastric and jejunoileal bypass procedures for morbid obesity. *Annals of Surgery,* 186: 500–509.

Güler A.K., Immenroth M., Berg T., Bürger T. & Gawad K.A. (2006). Evaluation einer neu konzipierten Operationsfibel durch den Vergleich mit einer klassischen chirurgischen Operationslehre. *Posterpräsentation auf dem 123. Kongress der Deutschen Gesellschaft für Chirurgie vom 02.–05. Mai 2006 in Berlin.*

Hanson D. (2004). Complications of weight loss surgery: implications for critical care nursing. Review. *Critical Care Nursing Clinics of North America,* 16: 553–558.

Hedberg J., Hedenström H., Nilsson S., Sundbom M. & Gustavsson S. (2005). Role of gastric acid in stomal ulcer after gastric bypass. *Obesity Surgery,* 15: 1375–1378.

Hell E., Miller K., Moorehead M.K., & Samuels N. (2000). Comparison of Standard Roux-en-Y Gastric Bypass, Vertical Banded Gastroplasty and Laparoscopic Adjustable Silicone Gastric Banding. *Obesity Surgery,* 10: 214–219.

Higa K., Ho T., Tercero F., Yunus T. & Boone K.B. (2011). Laparoscopic Roux-en-Y gastric bypass: 10-year follow-up. *Surgery for Obesity and Related Diseases,* 7: 516–525.

Higa K.D., Ho T. & Boone K.B. (2001). Laparoscopic Roux-en-Y gastric bypass: technique and 3-year follow-up. *Journal of Laparoendoscopic & Advanced Surgical Techniques,* 11: 377–382.

Higa K.D., Ho T. & Boone K.B. (2003). Internal hernias after laparoscopic Roux-en-Y gastric bypass: incidence, treatment and prevention. *Obesity Surgery,* 13: 350–354.

Immenroth M. (2003). *Mentales Training in der Medizin. Anwendung in der Chirurgie und Zahnmedizin.* Hamburg: Kovac.

Immenroth M., Bürger T., Brenner J., Kemmler R., Nagelschmidt R., Eberspächer H. & Troidl H. (2005). Mentales Training in der Chirurgie. *Der Chirurg* BDC, 44: 21–25.

Immenroth M., Eberspächer H., Nagelschmidt M., Troidl H., Bürger T., Brenner J., Berg T., Müller M. & Kemmler R. (2005). Mentales Training in der Chirurgie – Sicherheit durch ein besseres Training. Design und erste Ergebnisse einer Studie. *MIC,* 14: 69–74.

Immenroth M., Bürger T., Brenner J., Nagelschmidt R., Eberspächer H. & Troidl H. (2007). Mental Training in surgical education: a randomized controlled trial. *Annals of Surgery,* 245: 385–391.

Immenroth M., Eberspächer H. & Hermann H.D. (2008). Training kognitiver Fertigkeiten. In J. Beckmann & M. Kellmann (Hrsg.), *Enzyklopädie der Psychologie (D, V, 2). Anwendungen der Sportpsychologie* (119–176). Göttingen: Hogrefe.

Inabnet W.B., Quinn T., Gagner M., Urban M. & Pomp A. (2005). Laparoscopic Roux-en-Y gastric bypass in patients with BMI <50: a prospective randomized trial comparing short and long limb lengths. *Obesity Surgery,* 15: 51–57.

Leyba J.L., Llopis S.N., Isaac J., Aulestia S.N., Bravo C. & Obregon F. (2008). Laparoscopic gastric bypass for morbid obesity – a randomized controlled trial comparing two gastrojejunal anastomosis techniques. *Journal of the Society of Laparoendscopic Surgeons,* 12: 385–388.

Lotze R.H. (1852). *Medicinische Psychologie und Physiologie der Seele.* Leipzig: Weidmann'sche Buchhandlung.

Mason E.E. & Ito I. (1967). Gastric bypass in obesity. *Surgical Clinics of North America,* 47: 1345–1351.

Merkle E.M., Hallowell P.T., Crouse C., Nakamoto D.A. & Stellato T.A. (2005). Roux-en-Y gastric bypass for clinically severe obesity: normal appearance and spectrum of complications at imaging. *Radiology,* 234: 674–683.

Miller G.A. (1956). The magical number seven plus or minus two: some limits on our capacity for processing information. *Psychological Review,* 63: 81–97.

Näslund I. (1986). The size of the gastric outlet and the outcome of surgery for obesity. *Acta Chirurgica Scandinavica,* 152: 205–210.

Nguyen N.T., Longoria M., Welbourne S., Sabio A. & Wilson S.E. (2005). Glycolide copolymer staple-line reinforcement reduces staple site bleeding during laparoscopic gastric bypass: a prospective randomized trial. *Archives of Surgery,* 140: 773–778.

Nguyen N.T., Nguyen C.T., Stevens C.M., Steward E. & Paya M. (2004). The efficacy of fibrin sealant in prevention of anastomotic leak after laparoscopic gastric bypass. *Journal of Surgical Research,* 122: 218–224.

Olbers T., Björkman S., Lindroos A., Maleckas A., Lönn L., Sjöström L. & Lönroth H. (2006). Body composition, dietary intake, and energy expenditure after laparoscopic Roux-en-Y gastric bypass and laparoscopic vertical banded gastroplasty: a randomized clinical trial. *Annals of Surgery,* 244: 715–722.

Olbers T., Fagevik-Olsén M., Maleckas A. & Lönroth H. (2005). Randomized clinical trial of laparoscopic Roux-en-Y gastric bypass versus laparoscopic vertical banded gastroplasty for obesity. *British Journal of Surgery,* 92: 557–562.

Olbers T., Lönroth H., Fagevik-Olsén M. & Lundell L. (2003). Laparoscopic gastric bypass: development of technique, respiratory function, and long-term outcome. *Obesity Surgery,* 13: 364–370.

Patel R.Y., Baer J.W., Texeira J., Frager D. & Cooke K. (2009). Internal hernia complications of gastric bypass surgery in the acute setting: spectrum of imaging findings. *Emergency Radiology,* 16: 283–289.

Rogula T., Yenumula P.R. & Schauer P.R. (2007). A complication of Roux-en-Y gastric bypass: intestinal obstruction. *Surgical Endoscopy,* 21: 1914–1918.

SAGES Guidelines Committee. (2009). SAGES guideline for clinical application of laparoscopic bariatric surgery. *Surgery for Obesity and Related Diseases,* 5: 387–405.

Sapala J.A., Wood M.H., Sapala M.A., Schuhknecht M.P. & Flake T.M. Jr. (2001). The micropouch gastric bypass: technical considerations in primary and revisionary operations. *Obesity Surgery,* 11: 3–17.

Sauerland S., Angrisani L., Belachew M., Chevallier J.M., Favretti F., Finer N., Fingerhut A., Garcia Caballero M., Guisado Macias J.A., Mittermair R., Morino M., Msika S., Rubino F., Tacchino R., Weiner R. & Neugebauer E.A. [European Association for Endoscopic Surgery]. (2005). Obesity surgery: evidence-based guidelines of the European Association for Endoscopic Surgery (EAES). *Surgical Endoscopy,* 19: 200–221.

Sjöström L., Gummesson A., Sjöström C.D., Narbro K., Peltonen M., Wedel H., Bengtsson C., Bouchard C., Carlsson B., Dahlgren S., Jacobson P., Karason K., Karlsson J., Larsson B., Lindroos A.K., Lönroth H., Näslund I., Olbers T., Stenlöf K., Torgerson J. & Carlsson L.M. (2009). Effects of bariatric surgery on cancer incidence in obese patients in Sweden (Swedish Obese Subjects Study): a prospective, controlled intervention trial. *The Lancet Oncology,* 10: 653–662.

Sjöström L., Narbro K., Sjöström C.D., Karason K., Larsson B., Wedel H., Lystig T., Sullivan M., Bouchard C., Carlsson B., Bengtsson C., Dahlgren S., Gummesson A., Jacobson P., Karlsson J., Lindroos A.K., Lönroth H., Näslund I., Olbers T., Stenlöf K., Torgerson J., Agren G. & Carlsson L.M. (2007). Effects of bariatric surgery on mortality in Swedish obese subjects (Swedish Obese Subjects Study). *The New England Journal of Medicine,* 357: 741–752.

Søvik T.T., Taha O., Aasheim E.T., Engström M., Kristinsson J., Björkman S., Schou C.F., Lönroth H., Mala T. & Olbers T. (2010). Randomized clinical trial of laparoscopic gastric bypass versus laparoscopic duodenal switch for superobesity. *British Journal of Surgery,* 97: 160–166.

Steele K.E., Prokopowicz G.P., Magnuson T., Lidor A. & Schweitzer M. (2008). Laparoscopic antecolic Roux-en-Y gastric bypass with closure of internal defects leads to fewer internal hernias than the retrocolic approach. *Surgical Endoscopy,* 22: 2056–2061.

Sugerman H.J., Starkey J.V. & Birkenhauer R. (1987). A randomized prospective trial of gastric bypass versus vertical banded gastroplasty for morbid obesity and their effects on sweets versus non-sweets eaters. *Annals of Surgery,* 205: 613–624.

Keywords

Editors

Marc Immenroth, PhD

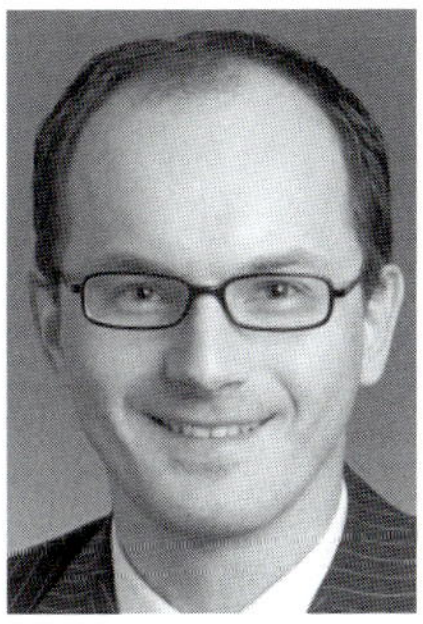

- Studied psychology (Diploma) and sports science (Master) in Heidelberg, Germany
- 1999–2006 Sports psychologist (including consultant to many top German athletes during their preparation for the World Championships and Olympics) and industrial psychologist (including consultant to Lufthansa Inc.)
- 2000 Research scientist at the University of Greifswald, Germany (Polyclinic for Restorative Dentistry and Periodontology)
- 2001–2004 Research scientist at the University of Heidelberg, Germany (Institute of Sports and Sports Science)
- 2002 Doctorate in psychology at the University of Heidelberg, Germany
- 2005–2006 Assistant lecturer at the University of Giessen, Germany (Institute of Sports)
- 2006–2008 Assistant professor at the University of Greifswald, Germany (Institute of Sports)
- 2006–2009 European Clinical Studies Manager at Ethicon Endo-Surgery (Europe) GmbH in Norderstedt, Germany
- 2009–2010 Marketing Manager and Sales Support at Ethicon Products, Johnson & Johnson MEDICAL GmbH in Norderstedt, Germany
- Since 2011 Senior Marketing Manager EP Germany & Plus Platform & Synthetic Absorbables D-A-CH, Johnson & Johnson MEDICAL GmbH in Norderstedt, Germany

Focus of Research and Work
- Mental training in sport, surgery and aviation
- Virtual reality in surgical education
- Coping with emotion and stress

Author of many scientific articles and textbooks on psychology, sports science and medicine

Jürgen Brenner, M.D.

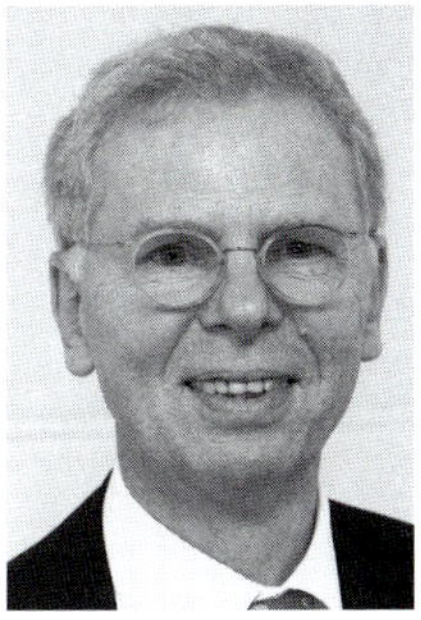

- Studied medicine in Hamburg, Germany
- 1972 Doctorate in medicine at the University of Hamburg, Germany
- 1972 Institute for Neuroanatomy, University of Hamburg, Germany
- 1974 Senior Resident at the Department of Surgery of the General Hospital Hamburg-Wandsbek, Germany
- 1981 Medical Director of the Department for Colorectal and Trauma Surgery at St. Adolf Stift Hospital in Reinbek, Germany
- 1987 Director for Surgical Research of Ethicon Inc. in Norderstedt, Germany
- 1989 Director of European Surgical Institute and Vice President Professional Education Europe of Ethicon Endo-Surgery (Europe) GmbH in Norderstedt, Germany
- 2004 Managing Director at Ethicon Endo-Surgery Germany in Norderstedt, Germany
- 2008–2011 Director of European Surgical Institute in Norderstedt, Germany
- Since 2011 Managing Director, Eric Krauthammer & Dr. Jürgen Brenner, Creative Team-Leadership

Assistants

Dr. Carl GmbH

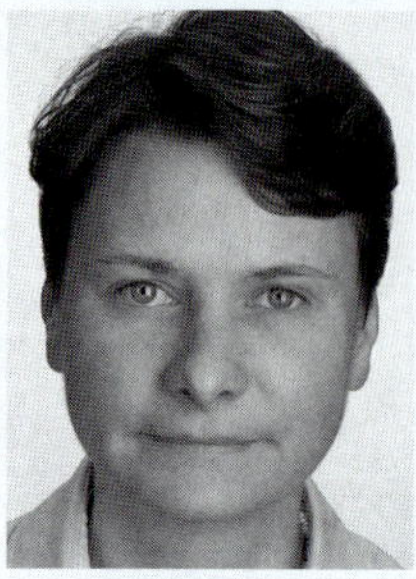

Indre Offermann, M.D.
Medical Writer

European Surgical Institute (ESI)

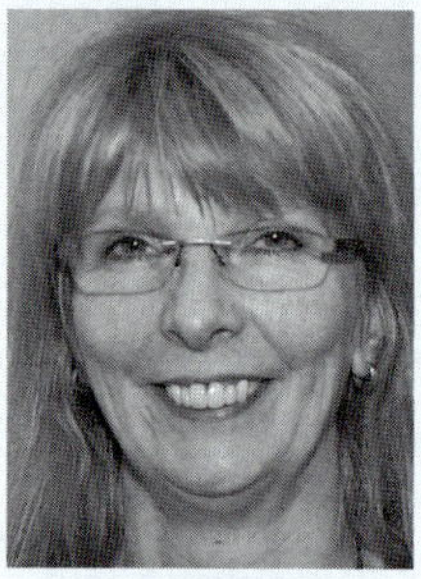

Maike Aukstinnis
Teamleader
Medical Training

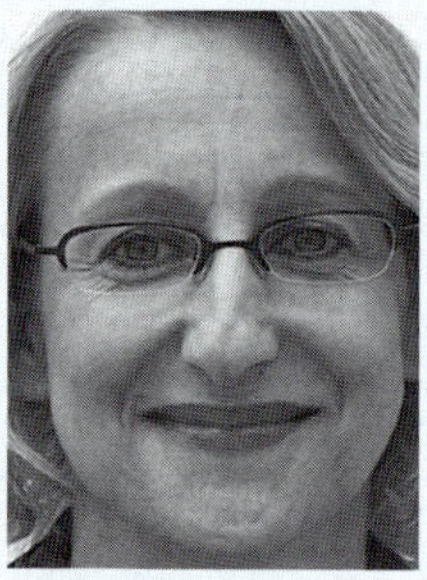

Astrid Künemund
Senior Manager
Medical Training

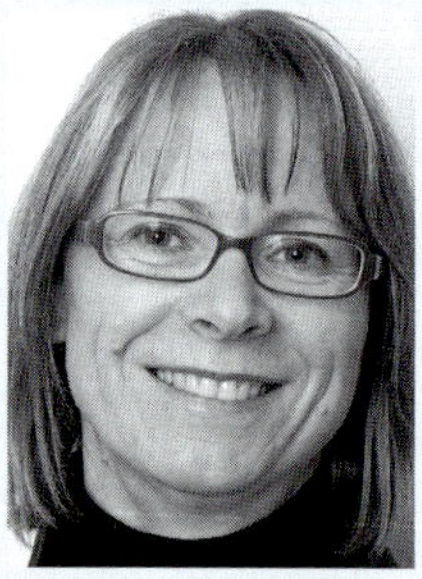

Annegret Röhling
Assistant ESI Director

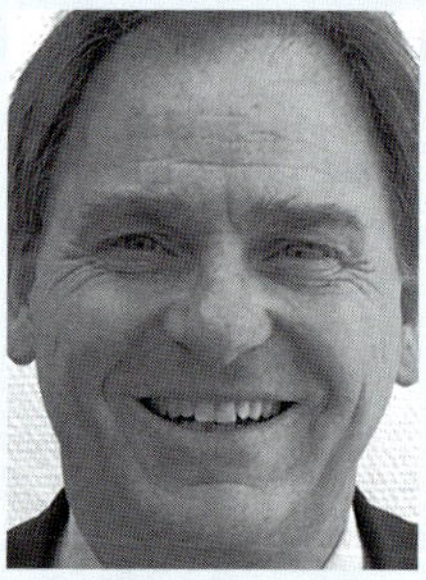

Detlev Ruge
Manager Event Technology

Ethicon Endo-Surgery Johnson & Johnson MEDICAL GmbH

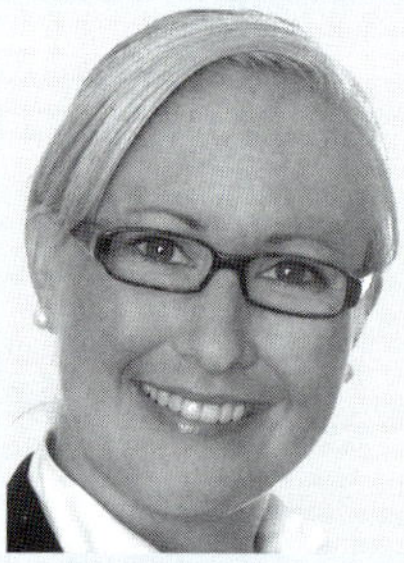

Ann-Katrin Güler, M.D.
Consultant Medical Products

Titles available

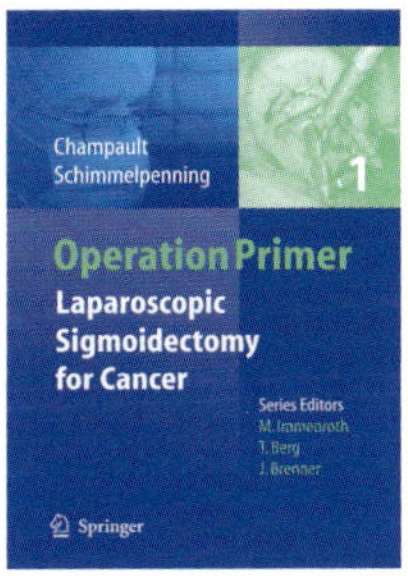

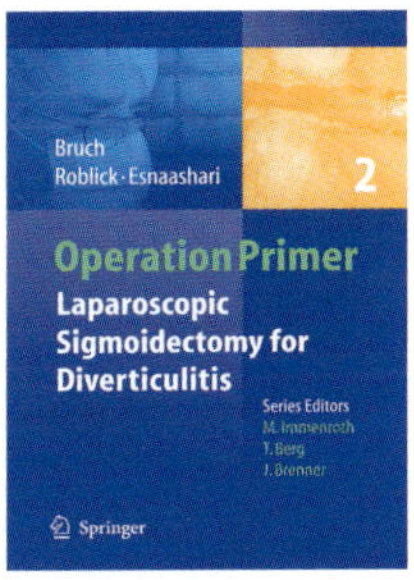

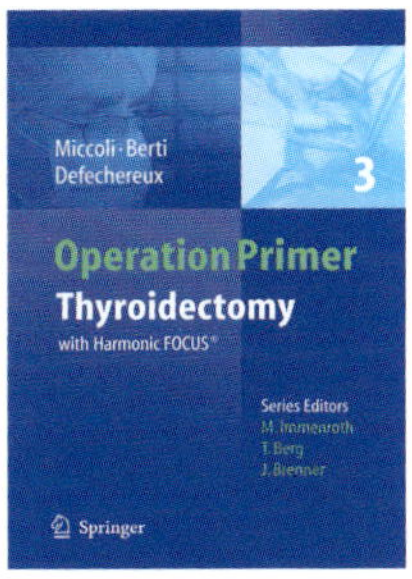

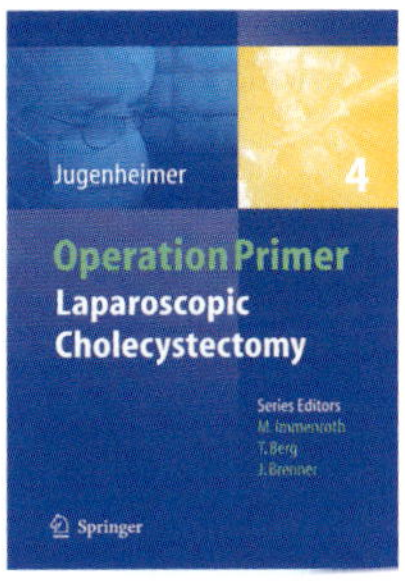

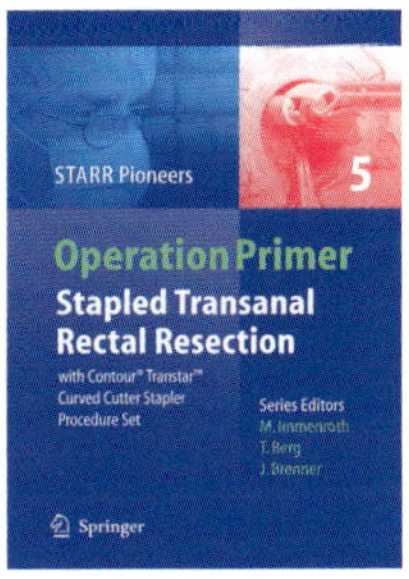

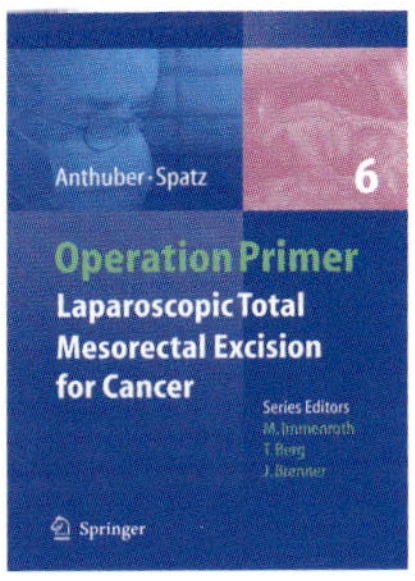

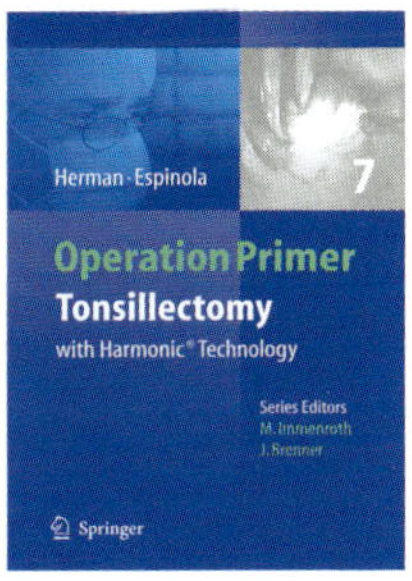

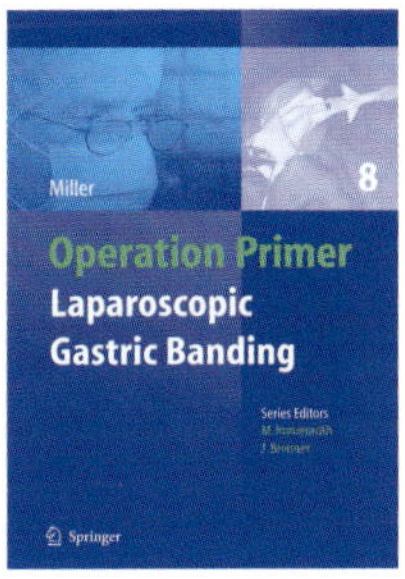

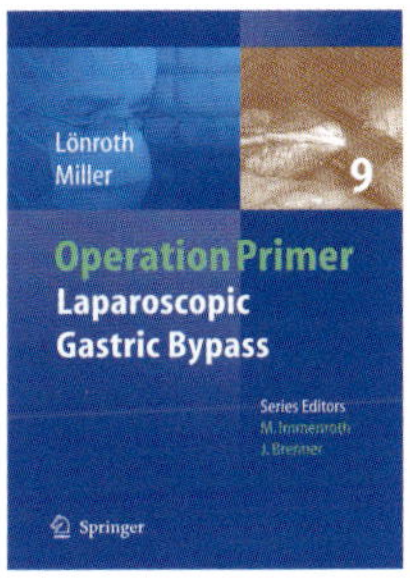

Volume 1:	Laparoscopic Sigmoidectomy for Cancer	ISBN 978-3-540-78453-1
Volume 2:	Laparoscopic Sigmoidectomy for Diverticulitis	ISBN 978-3-540-78451-7
Volume 3:	Thyroidectomy with Harmonic FOCUS®	ISBN 978-3-540-85163-9
Volume 4:	Laparoscopic Cholecystectomy	ISBN 978-3-540-92961-1
Volume 5:	Stapled Transanal Rectal Resection with Contour® Transtar™ Curved Cutter Stapler Procedure Set	ISBN 978-3-540-92958-1
Volume 6:	Laparoscopic Total Mesorectal Excision for Cancer	ISBN 978-3-642-04730-5
Volume 7:	Tonsillectomy with Harmonic® Technology	ISBN 978-3-642-12747-2
Volume 8:	Laparoscopic Gastric Banding	ISBN 978-3-642-19274-6
Volume 9:	Laparoscopic Gastric Bypass	ISBN 978-3-642-23001-1

Titles in preparation

Open Total Mesorectal Excision for Rectal Cancer

Laparoscopic Sleeve Gastrectomy

Video-assisted Thoracoscopic Lobectomy

Laparoscopic Hysterectomy

NOTES

NOTES